Health Care Finance
Basic Tools for Nonfinancial Managers

Judith J. Baker, PhD, CPA
Executive Director
Resource Group, Ltd.
Dallas, Texas

R.W. Baker, JD
Managing Partner
Resource Group, Ltd.
Dallas, Texas

JONES AND BARTLETT PUBLISHERS
Sudbury, Massachusetts
BOSTON   TORONTO   LONDON   SINGAPORE

World Headquarters

Jones and Bartlett Publishers
40 Tall Pine Drive
Sudbury, MA 01776
978-443-5000
info@jbpub.com
www.jbpub.com

Jones and Bartlett Publishers
Canada
2406 Nikanna Road
Mississauga, ON L5C 2W6
CANADA

Jones and Bartlett Publishers
International
Barb House, Barb Mews
London W6 7PA
UK

Copyright © 2004 by Jones and Bartlett Publishers, Inc.
Originally published by Aspen Publishers, Inc.© 2000.

LIBRARY OF CONGRESS CATALOGING-IN-PUBLICATION DATA
Baker, Judith J.
Health care finance: basic tools for financial managers/
Judith J. Baker, R.W. Baker
p. cm.
Includes bibliographical references and index.
ISBN 0-7637-3349-0
1. Health facilities—Finance Case studies. 2. Health facilities—Accounting Case studies. I. Baker, R.W. II. Title.
RA971.3.B353 1999
362.1'068'1—dc21
99-38261
CIP

PRODUCTION CREDITS
Publisher: Michael Brown
Production Manager: Amy Rose
Associate Editor: Chambers Moore
Associate Production Editor: Renée Sekerak
Production Assistant: Jenny L. McIsaac
Associate Marketing Manager: Joy Stark-Vancs
Manufacturing Buyer: Amy Bacus
Printing and Binding: PA Hutchison
Cover Printing: PA Hutchison

Printed in the United States of America
07 06 05 04 03   10 9 8 7 6 5 4 3 2 1

To the pioneers of management thought,
who laid the foundations we all build upon.

Table of Contents

Preface

Our world of work is divided into three parts: the health care consultant, the instructor, and the writer. Over the years, we have taught managers in seminars, in academic settings, and in corporate conference rooms. Most of the managers were midcareer adults, working in all types of health care disciplines. We taught them, and they taught us. One of the things they taught us was this: a nonfinancial manager pushed into dealing with the world of finance often feels a dislocation and a change of perspective, and that experience can be both difficult and exciting. We have listened to their questions and concerns as these managers grapple with this new world. This book is the result of their experiences, and ours.

The book is designed for use by a manager (or future manager) who does not have an educational background in financial management. It has long been our philosophy that if you can truly understand how a thing works—whatever it is—then you own it. This book is created around that philosophy. In other words, we intend to make financial management transparent by showing how it works and how a manager can use it.

USING THE BOOK

Users will find examples and exercises covering many types of health care settings and providers included. The case study of Metropolis Hospital System is woven throughout the book. Three mini-case studies are provided to give an even broader view of the subjects covered. "Progress Notes" set out learning objectives at the beginning of each chapter. An "Information Checkpoint" segment at the end of each chapter tells the user three things: information needed, where this information can be obtained, and how this information can be used. A "Key Terms" section follows the "Information Checkpoint." Each of these features displays its own quick-reference icon.

This book provides spreadsheet application templates for use with problems. The spreadsheet applications are available through a web site. Easy access to the web site is shown in

Appendix B, "Web-Based Learning Tools." For users who prefer a calculator, Appendix B provides guidance on where to obtain information on using a business analyst calculator. And for those users who choose neither a computer nor a calculator, instructions are set out so problems can also be worked by hand, with paper and pencil.

Acknowledgments

The book originated during the course of our activity-based costing seminars for Irwin Professional Seminars, when class members kept inserting finance questions into the sessions. The original concept for the book was clarified when Cleo Boulter, then Associate Professor at the University of Texas at Houston Center on Aging, recruited us to teach intensive finance sessions to her midcareer students, an arrangement that continued over a period of years. The needs of these students and their reaction to the material provided the initial core of the book's content.

Special thanks go to Craig Sheagren, Senior Vice President/CFO, McDonough District Hospital, Macomb, Illinois, and Nancy M. Borkowski, PhD, Professor, Department of Professional Management/Health Management, St. Thomas University, Miami, Florida, for their continued encouragement, information, suggestions, and assistance.

Many others contributed suggestions, recommendations, and information to help shape and refine the book. We thank:

Ian G. Worden, CPA, Regional Vice President of Finance/CFO, PeaceHealth, Eugene, Oregon

Robert Barker, Jr., CPA, Barker and Company, Dallas, Texas

Carol A. Robinson, Medical Records Director, Titus Regional Medical Center, Mt Pleasant, Texas

John Congelli, Vice President of Finance, Genesee Memorial Hospital, Batavia, New York

Charles A. Keil, Cost Accountant, Genesee Memorial Hospital, Batavia, New York

George O. Kimbro, CPA, CFO, Hunt Memorial Hospital District, Greenville, Texas

Bob Gault, Laboratory Director, Hunt Memorial Hospital District, Greenville, Texas

Ted J. Stuart, Jr., MD, MBA, Northwest Family Physicians, Glendale, Arizona

Mark Potter, EMS Director, Hopkins County Memorial Hospital, Sulphur Springs, Texas

and

Leonard H. Friedman, PhD, Assistant Professor, Coordinator, Health Care Administration Program, Oregon State University, Corvallis, Oregon

Patricia Chiverton, EdD, RN, Associate Dean, University of Rochester School of Nursing, Rochester, New York

Donna M. Tortoretti, RNC, Chief Operating Officer, Community Nursing Center, University of Rochester School of Nursing, Rochester, New York

Billie Ann Brotman, PhD, Professor of Finance, Department of Economics and Finance, Kennesaw State University, Kennesaw, Georgia

Health Care Finance Overview

CHAPTER 1

Background

PROGRESS NOTES

After completing this chapter, you should be able to

1. Understand the history of financial management.
2. Understand the basic concept of this book.
3. Discuss the three viewpoints of managers in organizations.

THE HISTORY

Financial management has a long and distinguished history. Consider, for example, that Socrates wrote about the universal function of management in human endeavors in 400 B.C. and that Plato developed the concept of specialization for efficiency in 350 B.C. And evidence of sophisticated financial management exists for much earlier times: the Chinese produced a planning and control system in 1100 B.C., a minimum-wage system was developed by Hammurabi in 1800 B.C., and the Egyptians and Sumerians developed planning and record-keeping systems in 4000 B.C.[1]

Many managers in early history discovered and rediscovered managerial principles while attempting to reach their goals. Because the idea of management thought as a discipline had not yet evolved, they formulated principles of management because certain goals had to be accomplished. As management thought became codified over time, however, the building of techniques for management became more organized. Management as a discipline for educational purposes began in the United States in 1881. On that date, Joseph Wharton created the Wharton School, offering college courses in business management at the University of Pennsylvania. It was the only such school until 1898, when the Universities of Chicago and California established their business schools. Thirteen years later, in 1911, 30 such schools were in operation in the United States.[2]

Over the long span of history, managers have all sought how to make organizations work more effectively. Financial management is a vital part of organizational effectiveness. This book's goal is to provide the keys to unlock the secrets of financial management for nonfinancial managers.

THE CONCEPT

A Method of Getting Money in and out of the Business

One of our colleagues, a nurse, talks about the area of health care finance as "a method of getting money in and out of the business." It is not a bad description. As we shall see, revenues represent inflow and expenses represent outflow. Thus, "getting money in" represents the inflow (revenues), whereas "getting money out" (expenses) represents the outflow. The successful manager, through planning, organizing, controlling, and decision making, is able to adjust the inflow and outflow to achieve the most beneficial outcome for the organization.

How Does Finance Work in the Health Care Business?

The purpose of this book is to show how the various elements of finance fit together: in other words, how finance works in the health care business. The real key to understanding finance is understanding the various pieces and their relationship to each other. If you, the manager, truly see how the elements work, then they are yours. They become your tools to achieve management success.

The health care industry is a service industry. It is not in the business of manufacturing, say, widgets. Instead, its essential business is the delivery of health care services. It may have inventories of medical supplies and drugs, but those inventories are necessary to service delivery, not to manufacturing functions. Because the business of health care is service, the explanations and illustrations within this book focus on the practice of financial management in the service industries.

VIEWPOINTS

The managers within a health care organization will generally have one of three views: (1) financial, (2) process, or (3) clinical. The way they manage will be influenced by which view they hold.

1. *The financial view.* These managers generally work with finance on a daily basis. The reporting function is part of their responsibility. They usually perform much of the strategic planning for the organization.
2. *The process view.* These managers generally work with the system of the organization. They may be responsible for data accumulation. They are often affiliated with the information system hierarchy in the organization.

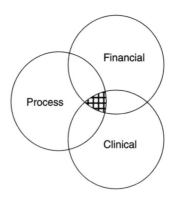

Figure 1–1 Three Views of Management within an Organization

3. *The clinical view.* These managers generally are responsible for service delivery. They have direct interaction with the patients and are responsible for clinical outcomes of the organization.

Managers must, of necessity, interact with one another. Thus, managers holding different views will be required to work together. Their concerns will intersect to some degree, as illustrated by Figure 1–1. The nonfinancial manager who understands health care finance will be able to successfully interpret and negotiate such interactions between and among viewpoints.

In summary, financial management is a discipline with a long and respected history. Health care service delivery is a business, and the concept of financial management assists in balancing the inflows and outflows that are a part of the business.

CHAPTER 2

Introduction to Health Care Finance

PROGRESS NOTES

After completing this chapter, you should be able to

1. Identify the four elements of financial management.
2. Understand the differences between the two types of accounting.
3. Identify types of organizations.
4. Understand the composition and purpose of an organization chart.

WHY MANAGE?

Business doesn't run itself. It requires a variety of management activities in order to operate properly.

THE ELEMENTS OF FINANCIAL MANAGEMENT

There are four recognized elements of financial management: (1) planning, (2) controlling, (3) organizing and directing, and (4) decision making. The four divisions are based on the purpose of each task. It should be noted that some authorities stress only three elements (planning, controlling, and decision making) and consider organizing and directing as a part of the controlling element.

This text recognizes organizing and directing as a separate element of financial management, primarily because such a large proportion of managers' time is taken up with performing these duties.

1. *Planning*. The financial manager identifies the steps that must be taken to accomplish the organization's objectives. Thus, the purpose is to identify objectives and then to identify the steps required for accomplishing these objectives.
2. *Controlling*. The financial manager makes sure that each area of the organization is following the plans that have been established. One way to do this is to study current reports and compare them to reports from earlier periods. This comparison often shows where the organization may need attention because that area is not effective. The reports used by the manager for this purpose are often called *feedback*. The purpose of controlling is to ensure that plans are being followed.
3. *Organizing and directing*. When organizing, the financial manager decides how to use the resources of the organization to most effectively carry out the plans that have been established. When directing, the manager works on a day-

to-day basis to keep the results of the organizing running efficiently. The purpose is to ensure effective resource use and provide daily supervision.

4. *Decision making.* The financial manager makes choices among available alternatives. Decision making actually occurs parallel to planning, organizing, and controlling. All types of decision making rely on information, and the primary tasks are analysis and evaluation. Thus, the purpose is to make informed choices.

THE ORGANIZATION'S STRUCTURE

The structure of an organization is an important factor in management.

Organization Types

Organizations fall into one of two basic types; they are either profit oriented or non–profit oriented. In the United States, these designations follow the taxable status of the organizations. The profit-oriented entities, also known as *proprietary organizations,* are responsible for paying income taxes. Proprietary subgroups include individuals, partnerships, and corporations. The nonprofit organizations do not pay income taxes.

There are two subgroups of nonprofit entities, voluntary and government. Voluntary nonprofits have sought tax-exempt status. In general, voluntary nonprofits are associated with churches, private schools, or foundations. Government nonprofits, on the other hand, do not pay taxes because they are government entities. Government nonprofits can be (1) federal, (2) state, (3) county, (4) city, (5) a combination of city and county, (6) a hospital taxing district (with the power to raise revenues through taxes), or (7) a state university (perhaps with a teaching hospital

affiliated with the university). The organization's type may affect its structure. Exhibit 2–1 summarizes the subgroups of both proprietary and nonprofit organizations.

Organization Charts

In a small organization, top management will be able to see what is happening. Extensive measures and indicators are not necessary because management can view overall operations. But in a large organization, top management must use the management control system to understand what is going on. In other words, to view operations, management must use measures and indicators because he or she cannot get a firsthand overall picture of the total organization.

As a rule of thumb, an informal management control system is acceptable only if the manager can stay in close contact with all as-

Exhibit 2–1 Types of Organizations

Profit Oriented—Proprietary
    Individual
    Partnership
    Corporation
    Other
Nonprofit—Voluntary
    Church Associated
    Private School Associated
    Foundation Associated
    Other
Nonprofit—Government
    Federal
    State
    County
    City
    City-County
    Hospital District
    State University
    Other

pects of the operation. Otherwise, a formal system is required. In the context of health care, therefore, a one-physician practice (see Figure 2–1) could use an informal method, but a hospital system (see Figure 2–2) must use a formal method of management control.

The structure of the organization will affect its financial management. Organization charts are often used to illustrate the structure of the organization. Each box on an organization chart represents a particular area of management responsibility. The lines between the boxes are lines of authority.

In the health system organization chart illustrated in Figure 2–2, the president/chief executive officer oversees seven senior vice presidents. Each senior vice president has vice presidents reporting to him or her in each particular area of responsibility designated on the chart. These vice presidents in turn have an array of other managers reporting to them at varying levels of managerial responsibility.

The organization chart also shows the degree of decentralization within the organization. Decentralization indicates the delegating of authority for decision making. The chart thus illustrates the pattern of how managers are allowed—or required—to make key decisions within the particular organization.

The purpose of an organization chart, then, is to indicate how responsibility is assigned to managers and indicate the formal lines of communication and of reporting.

TWO TYPES OF ACCOUNTING

Financial

Financial accounting is generally for outside, or third-party, use. Thus, financial accounting emphasizes external reporting. External reporting to third parties in health care includes, for example, government entities (Medicare, Medicaid, and other government programs) and health plan payers. In addition, proprietary organizations may have to report to stockholders, taxing district hospitals have to report to taxpayers, and so on.

Financial reporting for external purposes must be in accordance with generally accepted accounting principles. Financial reporting is usually concerned with transactions that have already occurred: that is, it is retrospective.

Managerial

Managerial accounting is generally for inside, or internal, use. Managerial accounting, as implied by its title, is used by managers. The planning and control of operations and related performance measures are common

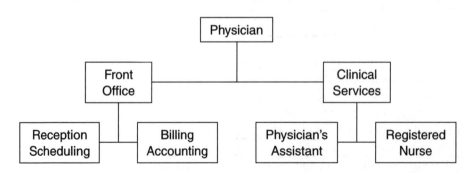

Figure 2–1 Physician's Office Organization Chart (Single Practitioner). Courtesy of Resource Group, Ltd., Dallas, Texas.

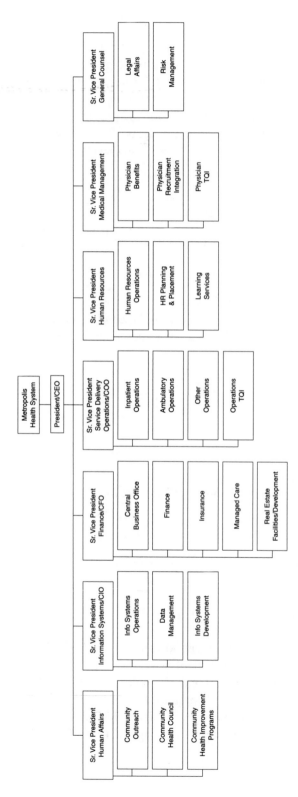

Figure 2–2 Health System Organization Chart. Courtesy of Resource Group, Ltd., Dallas, Texas.

day-by-day uses of managerial accounting. Likewise, the reporting of profitability of services and the pricing of services are other common ongoing uses of managerial accounting. Strategic planning and other intermediate and long-term decision making represent an additional use of managerial accounting.[1]

Managerial accounting intended for internal use is not bound by generally accepted accounting principles. Managerial accounting deals with transactions that have already occurred, but it is also concerned with the future, in the form of projecting outcomes and preparing budgets. Thus, managerial accounting is prospective as well as retrospective.

 ## INFORMATION CHECKPOINT

What Is Needed?	Reports for management purposes.
Where Is It Found?	With your supervisor.
How Is It Used?	To manage better.

What Is Needed?	Organization chart.
Where Is It Found?	With your supervisor or in the administrative offices.
How Is It Used?	To better understand the structure and lines of authority in your organization.

 ## KEY TERMS

Controlling
Decision Making
Financial Accounting
Managerial Accounting
Nonprofit Organization (also see *Voluntary Organization*)
Organization Chart
Organizing
Planning
Proprietary Organization (also see *Profit-Oriented Organization*)

 ## DISCUSSION QUESTIONS

1. What element of financial management do you perform most often in your job?
2. Do you perform all four elements? If not, why not?
3. Of the organization types described in this chapter, what type is the one you work for?
4. Have you ever seen your company's organization chart? If so, how decentralized is it?
5. If you receive reports in the course of your work, do you believe they are prepared for outside (third-party) use or for internal (management) use? What leads you to believe this?

CHAPTER 3

What Does the Health Care Manager Need To Know?

HOW THE SYSTEM WORKS IN HEALTH CARE

The information that you, as a manager, work with is only one part of an overall system. To understand financial management, it is essential to recognize the overall system in which your organization operates. There is an order to the system, and it is generally up to you to find that order. Watch for how the information fits together. The four segments that make a health care financial system work are (1) the original records, (2) the information system, (3) the accounting system, (4) and the reporting system. Generally speaking, the original records provide evidence that some event has occurred; the information

system gathers this evidence; the accounting system records the evidence; and the reporting system produces reports of the effect. The health care manager needs to know that these separate elements exist and that they work together for an end result.

THE INFORMATION FLOW

Structure of the Information System

Information systems can be simplistic or highly complex. They can be fully automated or semiautomated. And occasionally—even today—they can still be generated by hand and not by computer. (This last instance is becoming rare and can happen today only in certain small and relatively isolated health care organizations that are not yet required to electronically submit their billings.)

We will examine a particular information system and point out the basics that a manager should be able to recognize. Figure 3–1 shows information system components for an ambulatory care setting. This complex system uses a clinical and financial data repository; in other words, both clinical and financial data are fed into the same system. An automated medical record is also linked to the system. These are basic facts that a manager should recognize about this ambulatory information system.

11

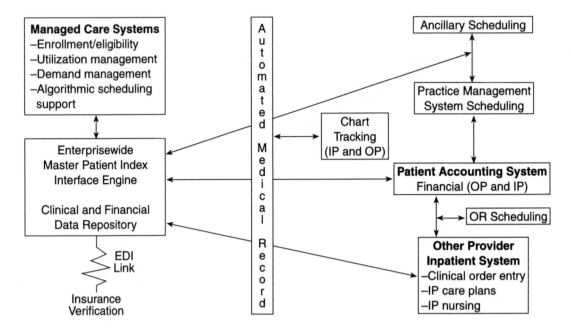

Figure 3–1 Information system components for an ambulatory care setting. OP, outpatient; IP, inpatient; OR, operating room.

In addition, the financial information, both outpatient and any relevant inpatient, is fed into the data repository. Scheduling-system data also enter the data repository, along with any relevant inpatient care plan and nursing information. Again, all these are basic facts that a manager should recognize about this ambulatory care information system.

These items have all been inputs. One output from the clinical and financial data repository (also shown in Figure 3–1) is insurance verification for patients through an electronic data information (EDI) link to insurance company databases. Insurance verification is daily operating information. Another output is decision-making information for managed care strategic planning, including support for demand, utilization, enrollment, and eligibility, plus some statistical support. The manager doesn't have to understand the specifics of all the inputs and outputs of this complex system, but he or she

should recognize that these outputs occur when this ambulatory system is activated.

Function of Flowsheets

Flowsheets illustrate, as in this case, the flow of activities that capture information.[1] Flowsheets are useful because they portray who is responsible for what piece of information as it enters the system. The manager needs to realize the significance of such information. We will give, as an example, obtaining confirmation of a patient's correct address. The manager should know that a correct address for a patient is vital to the smooth operation of the system. An incorrect address will, for example, cause the billing to be rejected. Understanding this connection between deficient data (e.g., a bad address) and the consequences (the bill will be rejected by the payer and thus not be paid) illustrates the essence of good financial management knowledge.

We can examine two examples of patient information flows. The first, shown in Figure 3–2, is a physician's office flowsheet for address confirmation. Note that four different personnel are involved in addition to the patient. This physician has computed the cost of a bad address as $12.30 to track down each address correction. He pays close attention to the handling of this information because he knows there is a direct financial management consequence in his operation.

The second example, shown in Figure 3–3, is a health system flowsheet for verification of patient information. This flowsheet illustrates the process for a home care system. Note that in this case the flow begins not with a receptionist, as in the physician office example, but with a central database. This central database downloads the information and generates a summary report to be reviewed the next day. Appropriate verification is then made in a series of steps, and any necessary corrections are made before the form goes to the billing department. The object of the flow is the same in both examples: that is, the billing must have a correct address to receive payment. But the flow is different within two different systems. A manager must understand how the system works to understand the consequences. Then good financial management can prevail.

BASIC SYSTEM ELEMENTS

To understand financial management, it is essential to decipher the reports provided to the manager. To comprehend these reports, it is helpful to understand certain basic system elements that are used to create the information contained in the reports.

Chart of Accounts—The Map

The chart of accounts is a map. It outlines the elements of your company in an orga-

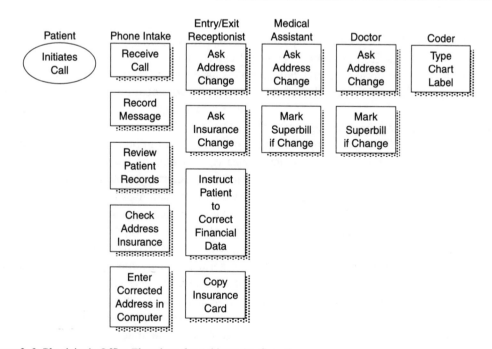

Figure 3–2 Physician's Office Flowsheet for Address Confirmation

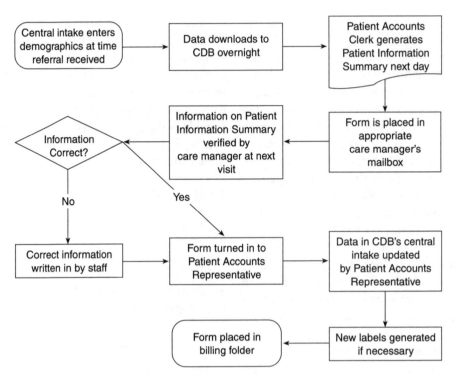

Figure 3–3 Health System Flowsheet for Verification of Patient Information

nized manner. The chart of accounts maps out account titles with a method of numeric coding. It is designed to compile financial data in a uniform manner that can be decoded by the user.

The groupings of accounts in the chart of accounts should match the groupings of the organization. In other words, the classification on the organization chart (as discussed in the previous chapter) should be compatible with the groupings on the chart of accounts. Thus, if there is a human resources department on your facility's organization chart, and if expenses are grouped by department in your facility, then we would expect to find a human resources grouping in the chart of accounts.

The manager who is working with financial data needs to be able to read and compre-

hend how the dollars are laid out and how they are gathered together, or assembled. This assembly happens through the guidance of the chart of accounts. That is why we compare it to a map.

Basic guidance for health care charts of accounts is set out in publications such as that of Seawell's Chart of Accounts for Hospitals.[2] However, generic guides are just that—generic. Every organization exhibits differences in its own chart of accounts that express the unique aspects of its structure. We will examine three examples to illustrate these differences. Remember, we are spending time on the chart of accounts because your comprehension of detailed financial data may well depend on whether you can decipher your facility's own chart of accounts mapping in the information forwarded for your use.

The first format, shown in Exhibit 3–1, is a basic use, probably for a smaller organization. The exhibit is in two horizontal segments, "Structure" and "Example." There are three parts to the account number. The first part is one digit and indicates the financial statement element. Thus, our example shows "1," which is for "Asset." The second part is two digits and is the primary subclassification. Our example shows "10," which stands for "Current Asset" in this case. The third and final part is also two digits and is the secondary subclassification. Our example shows "11," which stands for "Petty Cash—Front Office" in this case. On a report, this account number would probably appear as 1-10-11.

The second format, shown in Exhibit 3–2, is full use and would be for a large organization. The exhibit is again in two horizontal segments, "Structure" and "Example," and there are now two line items appearing in the Example section. This full-use example has five parts to the account number. The first part is two digits and indicates the entity designator number. Thus, we conclude that there is more than one entity within this system. Our example shows "10," which stands for "Hospital A." The second part is two digits and indicates the fund designator number. Thus, we conclude there is more than one fund within this system. Our example shows "10," which stands for "General Fund."

The third part of Exhibit 3–2 is one digit and indicates the financial statement element. Thus, the first line of our example shows "4," which is for "Revenue" and the second line of our example shows "6," which is for "Expense." (Note that the third part of this example is the first part of the simpler example shown in Exhibit 3–1.) The fourth part is four digits and is the primary subclassification. Our example shows "3125," which stands for

---

Exhibit 3–1 Chart of Accounts, Format 1

Structure		
X	XX	XX
Financial Statement Element	Primary Subclassification	Secondary Subclassification

Example		
1	10	11
Asset	Current Asset	Petty Cash— Front Office
(Financial Statement Element)	(Primary Subclassification)	(Secondary Subclassification)

Exhibit 3–2 Chart of Accounts, Format 2

Structure				
XX	XX	X	XXXX	XX
Entity Designator	Fund Designator	Financial Statement Element	Primary Subclassification	Secondary Subclassification

Example				
10	10	4	3125	03
Hospital A	General Fund	Revenue	Lab—Microbiology	Payer: XYZ HMO
10	10	6	3125	10
Hospital A	General Fund	Expense	Lab—Microbiology	Clerical Salaries
(Entity Designator)	(Fund Designator)	(Financial Statement Element)	(Primary Subclassification)	(Secondary Subclassification)

"Lab—Microbiology." The number "3125" appears on both lines of this example, indicating that both the revenue and the expense belong to Lab—Microbiology. (Note that the fourth part of this example is the second part of the simpler example shown in Exhibit 3–1. Note also that the simpler example used only two digits for this part but that this full-use example uses four digits.) The fifth and final part is two digits and is the secondary subclassification. Our example shows "03" on the first line, the revenue line, which stands for "Payer: XYZ HMO" and indicates the source of the revenue. On the second line, the expense line, our example shows "10," which stands for "Clerical Salaries." Therefore, we understand that these are the clerical salaries belonging to Lab—Microbiology in Hospital A. (Note that the fifth part of this example is the third and final part of the simpler example shown in Exhibit 3–1.) On a report, these account numbers might appear as 10-10-4-3125-03 and 10-10-6-3125-10. Another optional usage that is easier to read at a glance is 10104-3125-03 and 10106-3125-10.

Because every organization is unique and because the chart of accounts reflects that uniqueness, the third format, shown in Exhibit 3–3, illustrates a customized use of the chart of accounts. This example is adapted from a large hospital system. There are four parts to its chart of accounts number. The first part is an entity designator and designates a company within the hospital system. The fund designator two-digit part as traditionally used (see Exhibit 3–2) is missing here. The financial statement element one-digit part as traditionally used (see Exhibit 3–2) is also missing here. Instead, the second part of Exhibit 3–3 represents the primary classification, which is shown as an expense category ("Payroll") in the example line. The third part of Exhibit 3–3 is the secondary subclassification, representing a labor subaccount expense designation ("Regular per-Visit RN"). The fourth and final part of Exhibit 3–3 is another subclassification that indicates the department within the company ("Home Health"). On a report for this organization, therefore, the account number 21-7000-2200-7151 would indicate the home care services company's payroll for regular per-visit RNs in the home health department. Finally, remember that time spent understanding your own facility's chart of accounts will be time well spent.

Books and Records—Capture Transactions

The books and records of the financial information system for the organization serve to capture transactions. Figure 3–4 illustrates the relationship of the books and records to each other. As a single transaction occurs, the process begins. The individual transaction is recorded in the appropriate subsidiary journal. Similar such transactions are then grouped and balanced within the subsidiary journal. At periodic intervals, the groups of

---

Exhibit 3–3 Chart of Accounts, Format 3

Structure			
XX	XXXX	XXXX	XXXX
Company	Expense Category	Subaccount	Department
(Entity Designator)	(Primary Classification)	(Secondary Subclassification)	(Additional Subclassification)

Example			
21	7000	2200	7151
Home Care Services	Payroll	Regular per-Visit RN	Home Health
(Company)	(Expense Category)	(Subaccount)	(Department)

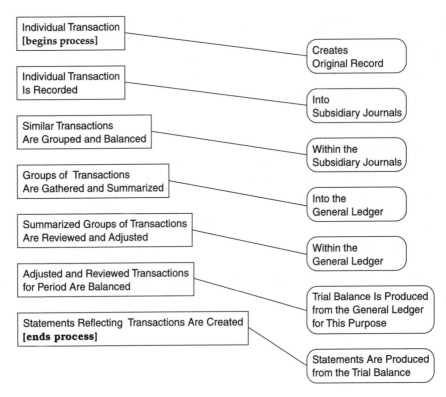

Figure 3–4 The Progress of a Transaction. Courtesy of Resource Group, Ltd., Dallas, Texas.

transactions are gathered, summarized, and entered in the general ledger. Within the general ledger, the transaction groups are reviewed and adjusted. After such review and adjustment, the transactions for the period within the general ledger are balanced. A document known as the trial balance is used for this purpose. The final step in the process is to create statements that reflect the transactions for the period. The trial balance is used to produce the statements.

All transactions for the period reside in the general ledger. The subsidiary journals are so named because they are "subsidiary" to the general ledger: in other words, they serve to support the general ledger. Figure 3–5 illustrates this concept. Another way to think of the subsidiary journals is to picture them as

feeding the general ledger. The important point here is to understand the source and the flow of information as it is recorded.

Reports—The Product

Reports are more fully treated in a subsequent chapter of this text (see Chapter 12). It is sufficient at this point to recognize that reports are the final product of a process that commences with an original transaction.

THE ANNUAL MANAGEMENT CYCLE

The annual management cycle affects the type and status of information that the manager is expected to use. Some operating infor-

THE BOOKS

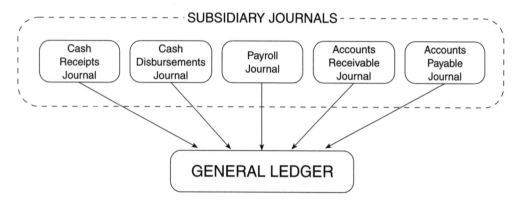

Figure 3–5 Recording Information: Relationship of Subsidiary Journals to the General Ledger. Courtesy of Resource Group, Ltd., Dallas, Texas.

mation is "raw"—that is, unadjusted. When the same information has passed further through the system and has been verified, adjusted, and balanced, it will usually vary from the initial raw data. These differences are a part of the process just described.

Daily and Weekly Operating Reports

The daily and weekly operating reports generally contain raw data, as discussed in the preceding paragraph. The purpose of such daily and weekly reports is to provide immediate operating information to use for day-by-day management purposes.

Quarterly Reports and Statistics

The quarterly reports and statistics generally have been verified, adjusted, and balanced. They are called *interim* reports because they have been generated sometime during the reporting period of the organization and not at the end of that period. Quarterly reports are often used as milestones by

managers. A common milestone is the quarterly budget review.

Annual Year-End Reports

Most organizations have a 12-month reporting period known as a fiscal year. A fiscal year therefore covers a period from the first day of a particular month (e.g., January 1) through the last day of a month that is one year, or 12 months, in the future (e.g., December 31). If we see a heading that reads "For the year ended June 30," we know that the fiscal year began on July 1 of the previous year. Anything less than a full 12-month year is called a "stub period" and is fully spelled out in the heading. If, therefore, a company is reporting for a three-month stub period ending on December 31, the heading on the report will read "For the three-month period ended December 31." An alternative treatment uses a heading that reads "For the period October 1 to December 31."

Annual year-end reports cover the full 12-month reporting period or the fiscal year.

Such annual year-end reports are not primarily intended for managers' use. Their primary purpose is for reporting the operations of the organization for the period to outsiders, or third parties.

Annual year-end reports represent the closing out of the information system for a specific reporting period. The recording and reporting of operations will now begin a new cycle with a new year.

INFORMATION CHECKPOINT

What Is Needed?	An explanation of how the information flow works in your unit.
Where Is It Found?	Probably with the information system staff; perhaps in the administrative offices.
How Is It Used?	Study the flow and relate it to the paperwork that you handle.

KEY TERMS

Accounting System
Chart of Accounts
General Ledger
Information System
Original Records
Reporting System
Subsidiary Journals
Trial Balance

DISCUSSION QUESTIONS

1. Have you ever been informed of the information flow in your unit or division?
2. If so, did you receive the information in a formal seminar or in an informal manner, one on one with another individual? Do you think this was the best way? Why?
3. Do you know about the chart of accounts in your organization as it pertains to information you receive?
4. If so, is it similar to one of the three formats illustrated in this chapter? If not, how is it different?
5. Do you work with daily or weekly operating reports? With quarterly reports and statistics?
6. If so, do these reports give you useful information? How do you think they could be improved?

PART II

Managerial Accounting and Financial Analysis

CHAPTER 4

Revenues (Inflow)

PROGRESS NOTES

After completing this chapter, you should be able to

1. Understand how receiving revenue for services is a revenue stream.
2. Recognize contractual allowances and discounts and their impact on revenue.
3. Understand the differences in sources of health care revenue.
4. See how to group revenue for planning and control.

OVERVIEW

Revenue represents amounts earned by an organization: that is, actual or expected cash inflows due to the organization's major business. In the case of health care, revenue is mostly earned by rendering services to patients. Revenue flows into the organization and is sometimes referred to as the *revenue stream.*

Revenue is generally defined as the value of services rendered, expressed at the facility's full established rates. For example, hospital A's full established rate for a certain procedure is $100, but Giant Health Plan has negotiated a managed care contract whereby the plan pays only $90 for that procedure.

The revenue figure—the full established rate—is $100. Note also that revenues can be received in the form of cash or credit. Most, but not all, health care revenues are received in the form of credit.

RECEIVING REVENUE FOR SERVICES

One way that revenue is classified is by whether payment is received before or after the service is delivered. The amount of revenue received for services is often influenced by this classification.

Payment after Service Is Delivered

The traditional payment method in health care is that of payment after service is delivered. Two basic types of payment after service is delivered will be discussed in this section: fee for service and discounted fee for service. One evolved from the other.

1. *Fee for service.* The truly traditional U.S. method of receiving revenue for services is fee for service. The provider of services is paid according to the service performed. Before the 1970s, with a very few exceptions, fee for service was the dominant method of payment for health services in the United States.[1]

2. *Discounted fee for service.* In this variation on the original fee for service, a contracted discount is agreed upon. The organization providing the services then receives a payment that is discounted in accordance with the contract. Sometimes the contract contains fee schedules. A large provider of services can have many different contracts, all with different discounted contractual arrangements. Many variations are therefore possible.

Payment before Service Is Delivered

Traditional payment methods in the United States have begun to give way to payment before service is delivered. There are multiple names and definitions for such payment. We have chosen to use a general descriptive term for payment received before service is delivered: *predetermined per-person payment.* The payment method itself and its rate-setting variations are discussed in this section.

1. *Predetermined per-person payment.* Payment received before service is delivered is generally at an agreed-upon predetermined rate. Payment therefore consists of the predetermined rate for each person covered under the agreement. Thus, the amount received is per-head or per-person count at a particular point in time.
2. *Rate-setting differences.* Different agreements can use varying assumptions about the group to be served, and these variations will affect the rate-setting process. Numerous variations are therefore possible.

Contractual Allowances and Other Deductions from Revenue

Revenues are recorded at the organization's full established rates, as previously dis-

cussed. Those amounts estimated to be uncollectible are considered to be deductions from revenues and are recorded as such on the books of the organization. (Note that, for purposes of the external financial statements released for third-party use, reported revenue must represent the amounts that payers [or patients] are obligated to pay. Therefore, the terms *gross revenue* and *deductions from revenue* will not be seen on external statements. The discussion that follows, however, pertains to the books and records that are used for internal management, where these classifications will be used.)

Contractual allowances are the difference between the full established rate and the agreed-upon contractual rate that will be paid. Contractual allowances are often for composite services. Take the case of hospital A as an example. As discussed in the overview to this chapter, hospital A's full established rate for a certain procedure is $100, but Giant Health Plan has negotiated a managed care contract whereby the plan pays only $90 for that procedure. The $10 difference between the revenue figure ($100) and the contracted amount to be paid by the plan ($90) represents the contractual allowance.

It is not uncommon for different plans to pay different contractual rates for the same service. This practice is illustrated in Table 4–1 which shows contractual rates to be paid for visit codes 99213 and 99214 for 10 different health plans. Note the variations in rates.

The second major deduction from revenue classification is an allowance for bad debts, also known as a provision for doubtful accounts. (Note once more that, for purposes of the external financial statements released for third-party use, the provision for doubtful reports must be reported separately as an expense item. The discussion that follows, however, still pertains to the books and records that are used for internal management, where

Table 4–1 Variations in Physician Office Revenue for Two Visit Codes

	Visit Codes	
Payer	99213	99214
FHP	$25.35	$35.70
HPHP	42.45	58.85
MC	39.05	54.90
UND	39.90	60.40
CCN	44.00	70.20
MAYO	45.75	70.75
CGN	10.00	10.00
PRU	39.05	54.90
PHCS	45.00	50.00
ANA	38.25	45.00

Rates for illustration only.

the classification of deductions from revenue will be used.) The allowance for bad debts is charged with the amount of services received on credit (recorded as accounts receivable) that are estimated to result in credit losses.

Beyond contractual allowances and a provision for bad debts, the third major deduction from revenue classification is charity service. Charity service is generally defined as services provided to financially indigent patients.

SOURCES OF HEALTH CARE REVENUE

Health care revenue in the United States comes from a variety of public programs (governmental sources) and private payers. The sources of health care revenue are generally termed *payers*. Payer mix—the proportion of revenues realized from the different types of payers—is a measure that is often included in the profile of a health care organization. For example, "Hospital A has a payer mix that includes 40 percent Medicare and 33 percent Medicaid" might be part of the profile.

Governmental Sources

The Medicare Program

Title XVIII of the Social Security Act is commonly known as Medicare. Actually entitled "Health Insurance for the Aged and Disabled," Medicare legislation established a health insurance program for the aged in 1965. The program was intended to complement other benefits (such as retirement, survivors', and disability insurance benefits) under other titles within the Social Security Act.

The Medicare program has two parts. One, known as Part A, is hospital insurance (HI) and is funded primarily by a mandatory payroll tax. The other part, known as Part B, is called supplementary medical insurance (SMI). SMI is voluntary and is funded primarily by insurance premiums (usually deducted from monthly Social Security benefit checks of those enrolled), supplemented by federal general revenue funds. Guidelines determine both the services to be covered and the eligibility of the individual to receive the services under the Medicare program. Medicare claims (billings) are processed by fiscal agents who act on behalf of the federal government. These fiscal agents are known as *intermediaries* and *carriers*. Intermediaries process the claims for Part A (HI) institutional services and outpatient claims for Part B (SMI). Carriers process the claims for Part B (SMI) physician and medical supplier services.

The Medicare program covers approximately 95 percent of the U.S. aged population along with certain eligible individuals receiving Social Security disability benefits.[2] Medicare is an important source of health care revenue to most health care organizations.

The Medicaid Program

Title XIX of the Social Security Act is commonly known as Medicaid. Medicaid legislation established a federal and state matching entitlement program in 1965. The program was intended to provide medical assistance to eligible needy individuals and families.

The Medicaid program is state specific. The federal government has established broad national guidelines. Each state has the power to set eligibility, service restrictions, and payment rates for services within that state. In doing so, each state is bound only by the broad national guidelines. Medicaid policies are complex, and there is considerable variation among states. The federal government is responsible for a certain percentage of each state's Medicaid expenditures; the specific amount due is calculated by an annual formula. The state pays the providers of Medicaid services directly. Thus, the source of Medicaid revenue to a health care organization is considered to be the state government's Medicaid program representatives.

The Medicaid program is the largest U.S. government program providing funds for medical and health-related services for the poor.[3] Therefore, although the proportion of Medicaid services within the payer mix may vary, Medicaid is a source of health care revenue in almost every health care organization.

Other Programs

There are numerous other sources of federal, state, and local revenues for health care organizations. Generally speaking, for most organizations none of the other revenue sources will exceed the Title XVIII and Title XIX programs just discussed. Other programs include the Department of Veterans' Affairs health programs, workers' compensation programs, and state-only general assistance programs (versus the federal-and-state jointly funded Medicaid program). Still other public programs are school health programs, public health clinics, maternal and child health services, migrant health care services, certain mental health and drug and alcohol

services, and special programs such as Indian health care services.

Managed Care Sources

In the 1970s, managed care began to appear in health care models in the United States. An all-purpose definition of managed care is: managed care is a means of providing health care services within a network of health care providers. The responsibility to manage and provide high-quality and cost-effective health care is delegated to this defined network of providers.[4] A central concept of managed care is the coordination of all health care services for an individual. In general, managed care plans receive a predetermined amount per member in premiums.

Types of Plans

The most prevalent type of managed care plan today is the health maintenance organization or HMO. Members enroll in the HMO. They prepay a fixed monthly amount; in return, they receive comprehensive health services. The members must use the providers who are designated by the HMO; if they go outside the designated providers, they must pay all or a large part of the cost themselves. The designated providers of services in turn contract with the HMO to provide services at agreed-upon rates. Several different forms of HMOs have evolved over time.

The preferred provider organization, or PPO, is a type of plan found across the United States. It consists of a group of providers called a panel. The panel members are an approved group of various types of providers, including hospitals and physicians. The panel is limited in size and generally has utilization review powers. If the patients in a PPO use health providers who are not within the PPO itself, they must pay a higher amount in deductibles and coinsurance.

Types of Contracts

In the case of an HMO, the designated providers of health services contract with the HMO to provide services at agreed-upon rates. The different types of HMOs—including the staff model, the group model, the network model, the point-of-service model, and the individual practice association (IPA) model—have various methods of arriving at these rates. A PPO contracts with its selected group, who are all participating payers, to buy services for its eligible beneficiaries on the basis of discounted fee for service. A large health care facility will have one or more individuals responsible for managed care contracting.[5]

Other Revenue Sources

A considerable amount of health care revenues is still realized from sources other than Title XVIII, Title XIX, and managed care:

- *Commercial insurers.* Generally speaking, conventional indemnity insurers, or commercial insurers, simply pay for the eligible health services used by those individuals who pay premiums for health care insurance. They do not tend to have a say in how those health services are administered.
- *Private pay.* This is payment by patients themselves or by the families of patients. Private pay is more prevalent in nursing facilities and in assisted living facilities than in hospital settings. Physicians' offices also receive a certain amount of private pay revenue.
- *Other.* Additional sources of revenue for health care facilities include donations received by voluntary nonprofit organizations and tax revenues levied by governmental nonprofit organizations.

Health care revenue is often reported to managers by source of the revenue. Table 4–2 presents such a revenue summary. This example covers all types of sources discussed in this section. Note that both dollar totals and proportionate percentages by source are reported.

GROUPING REVENUE FOR PLANNING AND CONTROL

Grouping revenue by different classifications is an effective method for managers to use the information to plan and to control. In the preceding paragraph, we have just seen revenue reported by source. Other classification examples will now be discussed.

Revenue Centers

A revenue center classification is one form of a responsibility center. In a responsibility center, the manager is responsible, as the name implies, for a particular set of activities. In the case of a revenue center, a particular unit of the organization is given responsibility for generating revenues to meet a certain target. Actually, the responsibility in the health care setting is more for generating volume than for generating a specific revenue dollar amount. (The implication is that the

Table 4–2 Sample Monthly Statement of Revenue by Source

Summary	Year to Date	%
Private revenue	$100,000	2.9
HMO revenue	560,000	16.7
Medicare revenue	1,420,000	42.4
Medicaid revenue	820,000	24.5
Commercial revenue	400,000	12.0
Other revenue	50,000	1.5
Total	$3,350,000	100.0%

volume will, in turn, generate the dollars.) Revenue centers tend to occur most often in special programs where volume is critical to survival of the program.

Care Settings

Grouping revenue by care setting recognizes the different sites at which services are delivered. The most basic grouping by care settings is inpatient versus ambulatory services. Exhibit 4–1, however, illustrates a six-way classification of care setting revenues within a health system. In this case, hospital inpatient, hospital outpatient, off-site clinic, skilled nursing facility, home health agency, and hospice are all accounted for. Note that a percentage is shown for each. This type of classification is useful for a brochure or a report that profiles the different types of health care services offered by the organization.

Service Lines

In traditional cost accounting circles, a product line is a grouping of similar products.[6] In the health care field, many organizations opt instead for "service line" terminology. A service line is a grouping of similar services. Strategic planning sometimes sets out service lines.

Hospitals

A number of hospitals have adopted the major diagnostic categories (MDCs) as service lines. One advantage of MDCs is that they are a universal designation in the United States. MDCs also have the advantage of possessing a standard definition. In another approach to service line classification, a hospital recently updated its strategic plan and settled on five service lines: (1) medical, (2) surgical, (3) women and children, (4) mental health, and (5) rehab (neuro ortho rehab) (see Figure 4–1).

Long-Term Care

A continuing care retirement community (CCRC) can use its various levels of care as a starting point. Thus, the CCRC usually has four service lines, listed in the descending order of resident acuity: (1) skilled nursing fa-

Exhibit 4–1 Revenues by Care Setting

42% Hospital Inpatient	38% Hospital Outpatient	4% Off-Site Clinic
8% Skilled Nursing Facility	6% Home Health Agency	2% Hospice

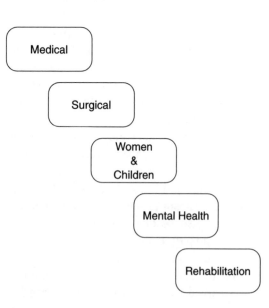

Figure 4–1 Hospital Service Lines. Courtesy of Resource Group, Ltd., Dallas, Texas.

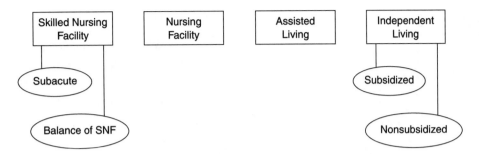

Figure 4–2 Long-Term Care Service Lines. Courtesy of Resource Group, Ltd., Dallas, Texas.

cility, (2) nursing facility, (3) assisted living, and (4) independent living. The skilled nursing facility provides services for the highest level of resident acuity, and the independent living provides services for the lowest level of resident acuity. One adjustment to this approach includes isolating subacute services from the remainder of skilled nursing facility services. Another adjustment involves splitting independent living into two categories, one for Housing and Urban Development (HUD)–subsidized independent housing and the other for private-pay independent housing. Figure 4–2 illustrates CCRC service lines by acuity level.

Home Care

Numerous categories of service delivery can be considered as "home care." A practical approach was taken by one home care en-

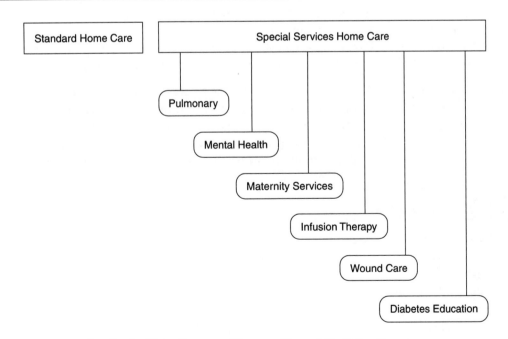

Figure 4–3 Home Care Service Lines. Courtesy of Resource Group, Ltd., Dallas, Texas.

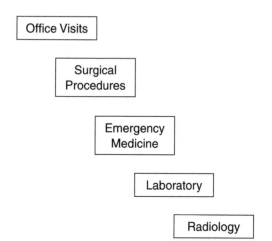

Figure 4–4 Physicians Group Service Lines. Courtesy of Resource Group, Ltd., Dallas, Texas.

tity—part of a health system—that defined its "key functions." Key functions can in turn be converted to service lines (see Figure 4–3).

Physician Groups

Service delivery for physician groups will vary, of course, with the nature of the group itself. A generic set of service lines is presented in Figure 4–4.

Other Designations

Other classifications may meet the needs of particular organizations. Columbia/HCA is now reported to classify its services in a disease management approach. The classification consists of eight disease management areas: (1) cancer, (2) cardiology, (3) diabetes, (4) behavioral health, (5) workers' compensation, (6) women's services, (7) senior care, and (8) emergency services.[7] Whatever classification is chosen, it must be consistent with the current structure of the organization.

 INFORMATION CHECKPOINT

What Is Needed?	A report that shows revenue in your organization.
Where Is It Found?	With your supervisor.
How Is It Used?	Examine the report to find various revenue sources; look for how the contractual allowances and discounts are handled on the report.
What Is Needed?	A report that groups revenue by some type of classification.
Where Is It Found?	With your supervisor, or in the information services division.
How Is It Used?	Examine the report to discover the methods that are used for grouping. You will probably find that these groupings are used for performance measures. They can also be used for control and planning.

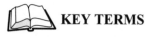 **KEY TERMS**

Discounted Fee for Service
Fee for Service
Managed Care
Medicaid Program
Medicare Program
Payer Mix
Revenue

DISCUSSION QUESTIONS

1. Does your organization receive revenue mainly in the form of payment after service is delivered or payment before service is delivered?
2. Why do you think this is so?
3. What do you believe the proportion of revenues from different sources is for your organization?
4. Do you believe that this proportion (payer mix) will change in the future? Why?
5. What grouping of revenue do you believe your organization uses (revenue centers, care settings, service lines, other)?
6. From your perspective, would there be a better grouping possible? If so, why do you think it is not used?

CHAPTER 5

Expenses (Outflow)

PROGRESS NOTES

After completing this chapter, you should be able to

1. Understand the distinction between expense and cost.
2. Understand how disbursements for services represent an expense stream (an outflow).
3. Follow how expenses are grouped in different ways for planning and control.
4. Recognize why cost reports have influenced expense formats.

OVERVIEW

Expenses are the costs that relate to the earning of revenue. Another way to think of expenses is as the costs of doing business. Just as revenues represent the inflow into the organization, so do expenses represent the outflow—a stream of expenditures flowing out of the organization. Examples of expenses include salary expense for labor performed, payroll tax expense for taxes paid on the salary, utility expense for electricity, and interest expense for the use of money.

In actual fact, expenses are expired costs—costs that have been used up, or consumed, while carrying on business. Revenues and expenses affect the equity of the business. The inflow of revenues increases equity, whereas the outflow of expenses decreases equity. In nonprofit organizations, the term is *fund balance* rather than *equity*. This is because a nonprofit organization, by its nature, is not in business to make a profit. Thus, it should not have equity. However, the principle of inflow and outflow remains the same. In the case of nonprofits, the inflow of revenues increases fund balance, and the outflow of expenses decreases fund balance.

Many managers use the terms *expense* and *cost* interchangeably. *Expense* in its broadest sense includes every expired (used-up) cost that is deductible from revenue. A narrower interpretation groups expenses into categories such as operating expenses, administrative expenses, and so on. *Cost* is the amount of cash expended (or property transferred, services performed, or liability incurred) in consideration of goods or services received, or to be received. As we have already said, costs can be either expired or unexpired. Expired costs are used up in the current period and are thus matched against current revenues. Unexpired costs are not yet used up and will be matched against future revenues.[1]

For example, an electric bill for $500 is recorded in the books of the clinic as an expense. The administrator sees the $500 as the cost of electricity for that month in the clinic. And the administrator is actually correct in seeing the $500 as a cost, because it has been used up (expired) within the month.

Confusion also exists in health care reporting over the term *cost* versus *charges*. Charges are revenue, or inflow. Costs are expenses, or outflow. Charges add; costs take away. Because the two are inherently different, they should never be intermingled.

DISBURSEMENTS FOR SERVICES

There are two types of disbursements for services:

1. *Payment when expense is incurred.* If an expense is paid for at the point where it is incurred, it does not enter the accounts payable account. In large organizations, it is relatively rare to see payments when expenses are incurred. The only place where this usually occurs is the petty cash fund.
2. *Payment after expense is incurred.* In most health care organizations expenses are paid at a later time and not at the point when the expense is incurred. If this is the case, the expense is recorded in accounts payable account. It is cleared from accounts payable when payment is made. One measurement of operations is "days in accounts payable," whereby the operating expenses for the organization are reduced to a rate per day and compared to the amount in accounts payable.

GROUPING EXPENSES FOR PLANNING AND CONTROL

Cost Centers

A cost center is one form of a responsibility center. In a responsibility center, the manager is responsible, as the name implies, for a particular set of activities. In the case of a cost center, a particular unit of the organization is given responsibility for controlling costs of the operations over which it holds authority. The medical records division is an example of a cost center. The billing and collection office might be another example. A cost center might be a division, an office, or an entire department, depending upon how the organization is structured.

In health care organizations, it is common to find departments as cost centers. This is often a logical way to designate a cost center because the lines of authority are generally organized by department. Cost centers can then be grouped into larger groups that have something in common. Within this method of grouping, the manager of a cost center may receive his or her own reports and figures but not those of the entire group. The director or officer that is in charge of all those particular departments receives the larger report that contains multiple cost centers. The chief executive officer receives a total report because he or she is ultimately responsible for overseeing the operations of all the cost centers involved in that segment of the organization.

Exhibit 5–1 illustrates this concept. It contains 20 different cost centers, all of which are revenue producing. The 20 cost centers are divided into two groups: nursing services and other professional services. There are five cost centers in the nursing services group, ranging from operating room to OB-nursery. There are 15 cost centers in the other professional services group. In the hospital that uses the grouping shown in Exhibit 5–1, however, not all of the 20 cost centers are departments. Some are divisions within departments. For example, EKG and EEG operate out of the same department but are two separate cost centers.

Exhibit 5–2 shows 11 different cost centers that are *not* directly revenue producing. (The

Exhibit 5–1 Nursing Services and Other Professional Services Cost Centers

Nursing Services Cost Center	
Nursing Services	
Routine Medical-Surgical	$390,000
Operating Room	30,000
Intensive Care Units	40,000
OB-Nursery	15,000
Other	35,000
Total	$510,000

Other Professional Services Cost Center	
Other Professional Services	
Laboratory	$220,000
Radiology	139,000
CT Scanner	18,000
Pharmacy	128,000
Emergency Service	89,000
Medical and Surgical Supply	168,000
Operating Rooms and Anesthesia	142,000
Respiratory Therapy	48,000
Physical Therapy	64,000
EKG	16,000
EEG	1,000
Ambulance Service	7,000
Substance Abuse	43,000
Home Health and Hospice	120,000
Other	12,000
Total	$1,215,000

partments.) The five cost centers in the support services group include one "general" cost center that contains administrative costs; the remaining four are related to employee salaries and wages. These four are insurance, social security taxes, employee welfare, and pension cost centers, all of which will probably be in the same department. It is the prerogative of management to set up cost centers specific to the organization's own needs and preferences. It is the responsibility of management to make the cost centers match the proper lines of authority.

Exhibit 5–2 illustrates two categories of health care expense: general services and support. A third related category is operations expense. An operations expense provides service directly related to patient care. Examples are radiology expense and drug expense. A general services expense provides services

Exhibit 5–2 General Service and Support Services Cost Centers

General Services Cost Center	
General Services	
Dietary	$97,000
Maintenance	92,000
Laundry	27,000
Housekeeping	43,000
Security	5,000
Medical Records	30,000
Total	$294,000

Support Services Cost Center	
Support Services	
General	$455,000
Insurance	24,000
Social Security Taxes	112,000
Employee Welfare	188,000
Pension	43,000
Total	$822,000

dietary department yields some cafeteria revenue, but that revenue is not central to the major business of the organization, which is to provide health care services.) The 11 cost centers are divided into two groups: general services and support services. The six cost centers in the general services group happen to all be departments in this hospital. (Other hospitals might not have security as a separate department. The other cost centers—dietary, maintenance, laundry, housekeeping, and medical records—would be separate de-

necessary to maintain the patient, but the service is not directly related to patient care. Examples are laundry and dietary. Support services expenses, on the other hand, provide support to both general services expenses and to operations expenses. A support service expense is necessary for support, but it is neither directly related to patient care nor is it a service necessary to maintain the patient. Examples of support services are insurance and payroll taxes.

Diagnoses and Procedures

It is common to group expenses by diagnoses and procedures for purposes of planning and control. This grouping is beneficial because it matches costs against common classifications of revenues. Much of the revenue in many health care organizations is designated by either diagnoses or procedures. One prevalent method groups costs into cost centers by major diagnostic categories (MDCs). The 23 MDCs serve as the basic classification system for diagnosis-related groups (DRGs). (Each DRG represents a category of patients. This category contains patients whose resource consumption, on statistical average, is equivalent. DRGs are part of the prospective payment reimbursement methodology.) Exhibit 5–3 provides a listing of the 23 MDCs.

How does the hospital use the MDC grouping? Exhibit 5–4 shows a departmental and cost center grouping in actual use. This hospital uses 27 cost center codes: the 23 MDCs plus four other codes ("Special Drugs," "HIV," "Unassigned," and "Outpatient"). The special drugs and HIV cost centers represent high-cost elements that management wants to track separately. "Unassigned" is a default category and should have little assigned to it. "Outpatient" is a separate cost center at the preference of management.

Exhibit 5–3 Major Diagnostic Categories

	Diseases and Disorders of the
MDC1	Nervous System
MDC 2	Eye
MDC 3	Ear, Nose, Mouth, and Throat
MDC 4	Respiratory System
MDC 5	Circulatory System
MDC 6	Digestive System
MDC 7	Hepatobiliary System and Pancreas
MDC 8	Musculoskeletal System and Connective Tissue
MDC 9	Skin, Subcutaneous Tissue, and Breast
MDC 10	Endocrine, Nutritional, and Metabolic
MDC 11	Kidney and Urinary Tract
MDC 12	Male Reproductive System
MDC 13	Female Reproductive System
MDC 14	Pregnancy, Childbirth, and the Puerperium
MDC 15	Newborns and Other Neonates with Conditions Originating in the Perinatal Period
MDC 16	Blood and Blood-Forming Organs and Immunological Disorders
MDC 17	Myeloproliferative and Poorly and Differentiated Neoplasms
MDC 18	Infections and Parasitic Diseases (Systemic or Unspecified Sites)
MDC 19	Mental Diseases and Disorders
MDC 20	Alcohol/Drug Use and Alcohol/Drug-Induced Organic Mental Disorders
MDC 21	Injuries, Poisoning, and Toxic Effect of Drugs
MDC 22	Burns
MDC 23	Factors Influencing Health Status and Other Contacts with Health Services

Exhibit 5–5 illustrates the grouping of costs for MDC 18 (Infectious Diseases). Eighteen is the hospital's departmental code, per Exhibit 5–4. The DRG classification, ranging from 415 to 423, appears in the next column. The description of the particular DRG appears in the third column, and the related cost appears in the fourth and final column. These costs can now be readily matched to equivalent revenues.

Outpatient services in particular are generally designated by procedure codes. Procedure codes, known as Physicians' Current Procedural Terminology (CPT) codes, are commonly used to group cost centers for outpatient services. (CPT codes represent a listing of descriptive terms and identifying codes for identifying medical services and procedures performed.) However, procedures can—and are—also used for purposes of grouping inpatient costs, generally within a certain cost center. A hospital example of reporting radiology department costs by procedure code appears in Table 5–1. In this example, the procedure code is in the left column, the description of the procedure is in the middle column, and the departmental cost for the particular procedure appears in the right column. These costs can now be readily matched to equivalent revenue.

Exhibit 5–4 Hospital Departmental Code List Based on Major Diagnostic Categories

1	Nervous System
2	Eye
3	Ear, Nose, Mouth, and Throat
4	Respiratory System
5	Circulatory System
6	Digestive System
7	Hepatobiliary System
8	Musculoskeletal System and Connective Tissue
9	Skin, Subcutaneous Tissue, and Breast
10	Endocrine, Nutritional, and Metabolic
11	Kidney and Urinary Tract
12	Male Reproductive System
13	Female Reproductive System
14	Obstetrics
15	Newborns
16	Immunology
17	Oncology
18	Infectious Diseases
19	Mental Diseases
20	Substance Use
21	Injury, Poison, and Toxin
22	Burns
23	Other Health Services
24	Special Drugs
25	HIV
26	Unassigned
59	Outpatient

Care Settings and Service Lines

Expenses can be grouped by care setting, which recognizes the different sites at which services are delivered. "Inpatient" versus "outpatient" is a basic type of care setting grouping. Or expenses can be classified by service lines, a method that groups similar services.[2]

If revenues are grouped by care setting or by service line, as discussed in the previous chapter, then expenses should also be grouped by these categories. In that way, matching of revenues and expenses can readily occur. A more detailed discussion of care settings and service lines, with examples, was presented in the preceding chapter.

Programs

A program can be defined as a project that has its own objectives and its own program indicators. Within management's functions of planning, controlling, and decision making, the program must stand on its own. A

Exhibit 5–5 Example of Hospital Departmental Costs Classified by Diagnoses, MDC, and DRG

	Hospital Departmental Code	*DRG*	*Description*	*Cost*
18	INFECTIOUS DISEASES	415	O/R—INFECT/PARASITIC DIS	$4,000
18	INFECTIOUS DISEASES	416	SEPTICEMIA)17	10,000
18	INFECTIOUS DISEASES	417	SEPTICEMIA 0–17	20,000
18	INFECTIOUS DISEASES	418	POSTOP/POSTTRAUMA INFECT	2,000
18	INFECTIOUS DISEASES	419	FEVER—UKN ORIG) 17W/C	3,000
18	INFECTIOUS DISEASES	420	FEVER—UKN ORIG) 17W/OC	6,000
18	INFECTIOUS DISEASES	421	VIRAL ILLNESS)17	4,000
18	INFECTIOUS DISEASES	422	VIR ILL/FEVER UNK 0–17	1,000
18	INFECTIOUS DISEASES	423	OT/INFECT/PARASITIC DX	3,000

program is often funded separately and for finite periods of time. For example, funds from a grant might fund a specific project for, say, three years. Often programs—especially those funded separately from the revenue stream of the main organization—have to arrange their expenses in a special format that is specified by the entity that provides the grant funds.

Program expenses should be grouped in such a way that they are distinguishable. Also, if such programs have been especially

Table 5–1 Example of Radiology Department Costs Classified by Procedure Code

Procedure Code	*Procedure Description*	*Department Cost*
557210	Ribs, Unilateral	$60,000
557230	Spine Cervical Routine	125,000
557280	Pelvis	33,000
557320	Limb—Shoulder	55,000
557360	Limb—Wrist	69,000
557400	Limb—Hip, Unilateral	42,000
557410	Limb—Hip, Bilateral	14,000
557430	Limb—Knee Only	62,000
	Total	$460,000

funded, the reporting of their expenses should not be commingled. An example of a program cost center is given in Exhibit 5–6. This cost center example has received special funds and must be reported separately, as shown.

COST REPORTS AS INFLUENCERS OF EXPENSE FORMATS

Cost reports are required by both the Medicare program (Title XVIII) and the Medicaid program (Title XIX). Every provider participating in the program is required to file an annual cost report. An array of providers who must file cost reports is illustrated in Table 5–2. The arrangement of expense headings on the cost reports has been consistent since the advent of such reports in 1966. Therefore, this standard and traditional arrangement has strongly influenced the arrangement of expenses in many health care information systems.

The cost report uses a method of cost finding. Its focus is what is called a cost center. The concept is not the same as the type of responsibility center "cost center" that has been discussed earlier in this chapter. Instead, the cost-finding "cost center" is, broadly speaking, a type of cost pool used in the cost-find-

Exhibit 5–6 Program Cost Center: Southside Homeless Intake Center

Program:	Southside Homeless Intake Center
Department:	Feeding Ministry
For the Month of:	January 2000
Raw Food	$14,050
Dietary Supplies	200
Paper Supplies	300
Minor Equipment	50
Consultant Dietician	50
Utilities	300
Telephone	50
Program Total	$15,000

Table 5–2 Selected Cost Report Forms

Type	Form
Hospital complex (includes all hospital-based facilities)	HCFA 2552
Skilled nursing facility	HCFA 2540
Home health agencies	HCFA 1728
Comprehensive outpatient rehabilitation facilities	HCFA 2088

ing process. The primary purpose of the cost pool/cost center in cost finding is to assist in allocating overhead.

The central worksheets for cost finding are Worksheet A, Worksheet B, and Worksheet B-1. Worksheet A contains the basic trial balance of all expenses for the facility. (Trial balances are discussed in a preceding chapter.) The beginning trial balance is reflected in the first three columns:

[Column 1]   [Column 2]   [Column 3]
"Salaries" + "Other"   = "Total"
(all other expenses)

The trial balance is grouped at the outset into cost center categories. The placement of these categories and their respective line items on the page stay constant throughout the flow of Worksheets A, B, and B-1. The cost centers are grouped into seven categories:

1. General service
2. Inpatient routine service
3. Ancillary service
4. Outpatient service
5. Other reimbursable
6. Special purpose
7. Nonreimbursable

The line items within these seven categories represent the long-lived traditional arrangement that has strongly influenced the arrangement of expenses in so many health care information systems.

 INFORMATION CHECKPOINT

What Is Needed?	A report that shows expense in your organization.
Where Is It Found?	With your supervisor.
How Is It Used?	Examine the report to find various types of expenses; look for how the expense flow is handled on the report.

What Is Needed?	A report that groups expenses by some type of classification.
Where Is It Found?	With your supervisor or in the information services division.

How Is It Used?   Examine the report to discover the methods that are used for grouping. You will probably find that these groupings are used for performance measures. They can also be used for control and planning.

 KEY TERMS

Cost
Diagnoses
Expenses
Expired Costs
General Services Expenses
Support Services Expenses
Operations Expenses
Procedures
Unexpired Costs

 DISCUSSION QUESTIONS

1. Have you worked with cost centers in your duties? If so, how have you been exposed to them?
2. Have you had to manage from a cost center type of report? If so, how was it categorized?
3. Do you believe that grouping expenses by diagnoses and procedures (based on type of services provided) is better to use for control and planning than grouping expenses by care setting (based on location of service provided)?
4. If so, why?
5. What grouping of expenses do you believe your organization uses (traditional cost centers, diagnoses/procedures, care settings, other)?
6. From your perspective, would there be a better grouping possible? If so, why do you think it is not used?

CHAPTER 6

Cost Classifications

PROGRESS NOTES

After completing this chapter, you should be able to

1. Distinguish between direct and indirect costs.
2. Understand why the difference is important to management.
3. Understand the composition and purpose of responsibility centers.
4. Distinguish between product and period costs.

DISTINCTION BETWEEN DIRECT AND INDIRECT COSTS

Direct costs can be specifically associated with a particular unit or department or patient. The critical distinction for the manager is that the cost is directly attributable. Whatever the manager is responsible for—that is, the unit, the department, or the patient—is known as a *cost object*.

The somewhat vague definition of a cost object is any unit for which a separate cost measurement is desired. It might help the manager to think of *cost object* as *cost objective* instead.[1] The important thing is that di-

rect costs can be traced. Indirect costs, on the other hand, cannot be specifically associated with a particular cost object. The controller's office is an example of indirect cost. The controller's office is essential to the overall organization itself, but its cost is not specifically—directly—associated with providing health care services. The critical distinction for the manager is that indirect costs usually cannot be traced but instead must be allocated or apportioned in some manner.[2] Figure 6–1 illustrates the direct-indirect cost distinction.

To summarize, it is helpful to recognize that direct costs are incurred for the sole benefit of a particular operating unit—a department, for example. As a rule of thumb, if the answer to the following question is "yes," then the cost is a direct cost: "If the operating unit (such as a department) did not exist, would this cost not be in existence?"

Indirect costs, in contrast, are incurred for the overall operation and not for any one unit. Because they are shared, indirect costs are sometimes called *joint costs* or *common costs*. As a rule of thumb, if the answer to the following question is "yes," then the cost is an indirect cost: "Must this cost be allocated in order to be assigned to the unit (such as a department)?"

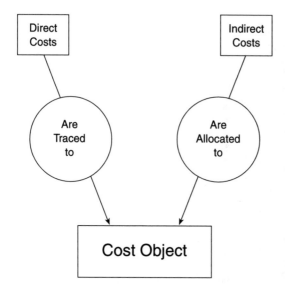

Figure 6–1 Assigning Costs to the Cost Object

EXAMPLES OF DIRECT COST AND INDIRECT COST

It is important for managers to recognize direct and indirect costs and how they are treated on reports. Two sets of examples will illustrate the reporting of direct and indirect costs. The first example concerns a radiology department; the second concerns a dialysis center.

Table 6–1 represents a report of two line items—direct costs and indirect costs—for a radiology department. The report concerns procedure nos. 557, 558, 559, 560, and 561 and a total. In this report, the manager can observe the proportionate differences between direct and indirect costs and can also see the differences among the five types of procedures.

Greater detail is provided to the manager in Table 6–2, which presents the method of allocating indirect costs and the result of such allocation. Managers should notice that the "totals" line carries forward and becomes the "indirect cost" line in Table 6–1. The purpose of the report in Table 6–2 is to reveal details that support the main report in Table 6–1. Thus, this report showing allocation of indirect costs is considered a subsidiary report because it is supporting, or subsidiary to, the preceding main report. This use of one or more supporting reports to reveal details behind the main report is quite common in managerial reports. The allocation of indirect costs subsidiary report contains quite a lot of information. It shows what line items (transporters, receptionists, etc.) are contained in the $1,267,000 total. It shows how each line

Table 6–1 Example of Radiology Departments Direct and Indirect Cost Totals

Dept: Radiology—Diagnostic
Cost Summary—Year to Date November 1999

Indirect Cost Centers	CC #557 Diagnostic Radiology	CC #558 Ultra- sound	CC #559 Nuclear Medicine	CC #560 CT Scan	CC #561 Radiation Therapy	Total
Direct costs	$1,000,000	$600,000	$1,200,000	$1,800,000	$1,400,000	$6,000,000
Indirect costs*	300,000	195,375	221,500	338,500	211,625	1,267,000
Totals	$1,300,000	$795,375	$1,421,500	$2,138,500	$1,611,625	$7,267,000

*See Table 6–2 for cost allocation detail.

Source: Adapted from A. Baptist, A General Approach to Costing Procedures in Ancillary Departments, *Topics in Health Care Financing,* Vol. 13, No. 4, p. 36, © 1987, Aspen Publishers, Inc.

Table 6-2 Example of Indirect Costs Allocated to Radiology Departments

Dept: Radiology—Diagnostic
Cost Summary—Year to Date November 1999

Indirect Cost Centers	Total Indirect Costs	Allocation Basis	CC #557 Diagnostic Radiology	CC #558 Ultrasound	CC #559 Nuclear Medicine	CC #560 CT Scan	CC #561 Radiation Therapy	Total
Transporters	$550,000	A	$110,000	$132,000	$88,000	$154,000	$66,000	$550,000
Receptionists	360,000	B	60,000	36,000	72,000	108,000	84,000	360,000
File room clerks	117,000	C	90,000	3,375	13,500	4,500	5,625	117,000
Managers	240,000	B	40,000	24,000	48,000	72,000	56,000	240,000
Totals	$1,267,000		$300,000	$195,375	$221,500	$338,500	$211,625	$1,267,000

Allocation Basis:

A. Volumes	100,000	120,000	80,000	140,000	60,000	500,000
B. Direct costs	$1,000,000	$600,000	$1,200,000	$1,800,000	$1,400,000	$6,000,000
C. Number of films	400,000	15,000	60,000	20,000	25,000	520,000

Source: Adapted from A. Baptist, A General Approach to Costing Procedures in Ancillary Departments, *Topics in Health Care Financing*, Vol. 13, No. 4, p. 36, © 1987, Aspen Publishers, Inc.

item is allocated across the five separate procedures. And it shows how each line item was allocated; see the "Allocation Basis" column containing codes of A, B, C, and D. Then see the box below with the allocation basis set out for type (volumes/direct costs/number of films) and for resulting allocation of each across the five procedures. This set of tables is worthy of further study by the manager.

Exhibit 6–1 sets out the direct costs for a freestanding dialysis center. These costs, as direct costs, are what the organization's managers believe can be traced to the specific operation of the freestanding center. Exhibit 6–2 sets out the indirect costs for a freestanding dialysis center. These costs are what the organization's managers believe are not directly attributable to the specific operation of the freestanding center. The decisions about what will and what will not be considered di-

rect or indirect costs will almost always have been made for the manager.[3] What is important is that the manager understand two things: first, why this is so, and second, how the relationship between the two works. Remember the rule of thumb discussed earlier in this chapter. If the answer to the following question is "yes," then the cost is a direct cost: "If the operating unit (such as a department) did not exist, would this cost not be in existence?"

RESPONSIBILITY CENTERS

In a previous chapter, we discussed revenue centers, whereby managers are responsible for generating revenue (or volume). We also previously discussed cost centers, whereby managers are responsible for managing and controlling cost. The responsibility center makes a manager responsible for both the revenue/volume (inflow) side and the expense (outflow) side of a department, division, unit, or program. In other words, the manager is responsible for generating revenue/volume and for controlling costs. Another term for responsibility center is *profit center*.

We will examine the type of information a manager receives about his or her own responsibility center by reviewing the Westside Center operations. Westside Center offers

Exhibit 6–2 Example of Freestanding Dialysis Center Indirect Costs

Indirect Costs	
Facility costs	$300,000
Administrative costs	300,000
Total indirect costs	$600,000

Courtesy of Resource Group, Ltd., Dallas, Texas.

Exhibit 6–1 Example of Freestanding Dialysis Center Direct Costs

Salaries and fringe benefits	$500,000
Salaries—other professional	40,000
Medical director	40,000
Medical supplies	550,000
Pharmacy	1,130,000
Dialysis center equipment depreciation	80,000
Utilities	80,000
Housekeeping and laundry	20,000
Property taxes	40,000
Other supplies and costs	20,000
Total direct costs	$2,500,000

Source: Adapted from D.A. West, T.D. West, and P.J. Malone, Managing Capital and Administrative (Indirect) Costs to Achieve Strategic Objectives: The Dialysis Clinic versus the Outpatient Clinic, *Journal of Health Care Finance,* Vol. 25, No. 2, p. 24, © 1998, Aspen Publishers, Inc.

two basic types of services: an ambulatory surgery center and a rehabilitation center. The management of Westside is overseen by Bill, the director. The ambulatory surgery center is managed by Joe. The rehabilitation center is managed by Bonnie. Denise, a part-time radiologist, provides radiology services on an as-needed basis. Joe, Bonnie and Denise, the managers, all report to Bill, the director. Figure 6–2 illustrates the managerial relationships.

To restate the relationships shown in Figure 6–2, Joe manages a responsibility center for ambulatory surgery services. Bonnie manages a responsibility center for rehabilitation services. These services represent the business of Westside Center. Denise manages the radiology services, but this is not a responsibility center in the Westside organization. Instead, it is a support center. Bill, the director, manages a bigger responsibility center that includes all of the functions just described plus the general and administrative support center.

Bill, the director, receives a managerial report shown in Exhibit 6–3. Bill's Director's Summary contains the data for the entire Westside operation.

Exhibit 6–3 Director's Summary of Westside ASC and Rehab Responsibility Center

ASC R/C Surplus	$70,000.00
Rehab R/C Surplus	85,000.00
Less G&A Support Ctr	(80,000.00)
Less Radiology Support Ctr	(20,000.00)
Net Surplus	$55,000.00

Courtesy of Resource Group, Ltd., Dallas, Texas.

Figure 6–3 illustrates the reports received by each manager at Westside. Joe's report for the ambulatory surgery center is at the top right of Figure 6–3. His report shows the controllable revenues he is responsible for ($225,000), less the controllable expenses he is responsible for ($150,000). The difference is labeled "ASC Responsibility Center Surplus" on his report. The surplus amounts to $70,000 ($225,000 minus $150,000).

Bonnie's report for the rehabilitation center is the second report on the right of Figure 6–3. Her report shows the controllable revenues she is responsible for ($300,000), less

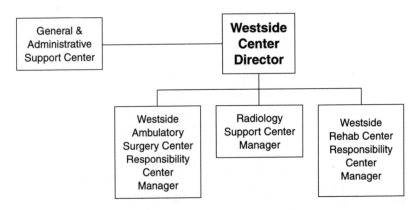

Figure 6–2 Lines of Managerial Responsibility at Westside Center. Courtesy of Resource Group, Ltd., Dallas, Texas.

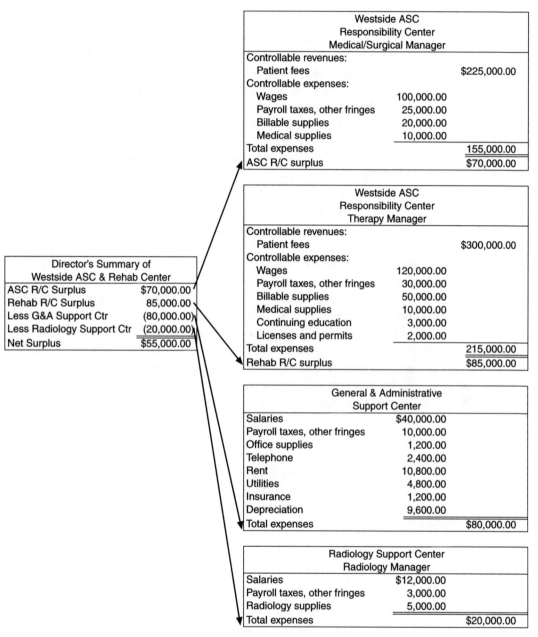

Figure 6–3 Westside Costs by Responsibility Center. Courtesy of Resource Group, Ltd., Dallas, Texas.

the controllable expenses she is responsible for ($215,000). The difference is labeled "Rehab Responsibility Center Surplus" on her report. The surplus amounts to $85,000 ($300,000 minus $215,000).

Denise's report for radiology services is at the bottom right of Figure 6–3. Her report shows the controllable expenses she is responsible for, which amount to $20,000. Her report shows only expenses because it is a support center, not a responsibility center. Therefore, Denise is responsible for expenses but not for revenue/volume.

Bill, the director, receives a report for the general and administrative (G&A) expenses, as shown second from the bottom right of Figure 6–3. This report shows the G&A controllable expenses Bill himself is responsible for at Westside, which amount to $80,000. The G&A report shows only expenses because it also is a support center, not a responsibility center. Therefore, Bill is responsible for expenses but not for revenue/volume in the case of G&A.

However, Bill is also responsible for the entire Westside operation. That is, the overall Westside operation is his responsibility center. Therefore, Bill's Director's Summary, reproduced on the left side of Figure 6–3, contains the results of both responsibility centers and both support centers. The surplus figures from Joe and Bonnie's reports are positive figures of $70,000 and $85,000, respectively. The expense-only figures from Bill's G&A support center report and from Denise's radiology support center report are negative figures of $80,000 and $20,000, respectively. Therefore, to find the result of operations for Bill's entire Westside operation, the $80,000 and the $20,000 expense figures are subtracted from the surplus figures to arrive at a net surplus for Westside of $55,000.

Although the lines of managerial responsibility will vary in other organizations, the relationships between and among responsibility centers, support centers, and overall supervision will remain as shown in this example.

DISTINCTION BETWEEN PRODUCT AND PERIOD COSTS

Product costs is a term that was originally associated with manufacturing rather than with services. The concept of product costs assumes that a product has been manufactured and placed into inventory while waiting to be sold. Then, whenever that product is sold, the product is matched with revenue and recognized as a cost. Thus *cost of sales* is the common usage for manufacturing firms. (The concept of matching revenues and expenses has been discussed in a preceding chapter.)

Period costs, in the original manufacturing interpretation, are not connected with the manufacturing process. They are matched with revenue on the basis of the period during which the cost is incurred (thus *period costs*). The term comes from the span of time in which matching occurs, known as *time period*.

Service organizations have no manufacturing process as such. The business of health care service organizations is service delivery, not the manufacturing of products. Although the overall concept of product versus period cost is not as vital to service delivery, the distinction remains important for managers in health care to know.

In health care organizations, product cost can be viewed as traceable to the cost object of the department, division, or unit. A period cost is not traceable in this manner. Another way to view this distinction is to think of product costs as those costs necessary to actually deliver the service, whereas period costs are costs necessary to support the existence of the organization itself.

One final note: medical supply and pharmacy departments do have inventories on hand. In their case, a product is purchased (rather than manufactured) and placed into inventory while waiting to be dispensed. Then, whenever that product is dispensed, the product is matched with revenue and recognized as a cost of providing the service to the patient. Therefore, the product cost concept is important to managers of departments that hold a significant amount of inventory.

INFORMATION CHECKPOINT

What Is Needed?   Example of a management report that uses direct/indirect cost.
Where Is It Found?   With your supervisor, in administration, or in information services.
How Is It Used?   To track operations directly associated with the unit.

What Is Needed?   Example of a management report that uses responsibility centers.
Where Is It Found?   With your supervisor, in administration, or in information services.
How Is It Used?   To reflect operations that a manager is specifically responsible for
                         and to measure those operations for planning and control.

 KEY TERMS

Cost Object
Direct Cost
Indirect Cost
Joint Cost
Responsibility Centers

 DISCUSSION QUESTIONS

1. In your own workplace, can you give a good example of a direct cost? An indirect cost?
2. What is the difference?
3. Does your organization use responsibility centers?
4. If not, do you think they should? Why?
5. If so, do you believe the responsibility centers operate properly? Would you make changes? Why?

CHAPTER 7

Cost Behavior and
Break-Even Analysis

DISTINCTION BETWEEN FIXED, VARIABLE, AND SEMIVARIABLE COSTS

This chapter emphasizes the distinction between fixed, variable, and semivariable costs because this knowledge is a basic working tool in financial management. The manager needs to know the difference between fixed and variable costs to compute contribution margins and break-even points. The manager also needs to know about semivariable costs to make good decisions about how to treat these costs.

Fixed costs are costs that do not vary in total when activity levels (or volume) of operations change. This concept is illustrated in Figure 7–1. The horizontal axis of the graph shows number of residents in the Jones Group Home, and the vertical axis shows total monthly fixed cost in dollars. In this graph, the total monthly fixed cost for the group home is $3,000, and that amount does not change, whether the number of residents (the activity level or volume) is low or high. A good example of a fixed cost is rent expense. Rent would not vary whether the home was almost full or almost empty; thus, rent is a fixed cost.

Variable costs, on the other hand, are costs that vary in direct proportion to changes in activity levels (or volume) of operations. This concept is illustrated in Figure 7–2. The horizontal axis of the graph shows number of residents in the Jones Group Home, and the vertical axis shows total monthly variable cost in dollars. In this graph, the monthly variable cost for the group home changes proportionately with the number of residents (the activity level or volume) in the home. A good example of a variable cost is food for the group home residents. Food would vary directly depending on the number of individuals in residence; thus, food is a variable cost.

Semivariable costs vary when the activity levels (or volume) of operations change, but

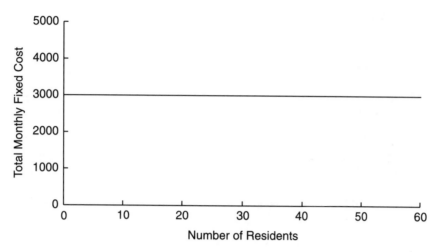

Figure 7–1 Fixed Cost—Jones Group Home

not in direct proportion. The most frequent pattern of semivariable costs is the step pattern, where the semivariable cost rises, flattens out for a bit, then rises again. The step pattern of semivariable costs is illustrated in Figure 7–3. The horizontal axis of the graph shows number of residents in the Jones Group Home, and the vertical axis shows total monthly semivariable cost. In this graph, the behavior of the cost line resembles stair steps: thus, the "step pattern" name for this configuration. The most common example of a semivariable expense in health care is supervisors' salaries. A single supervisor, for example, can perform adequately over a range of rises in activity levels (or volume). When another supervisor has to be added, the rise in the step pattern occurs.

It is important to know, however, that there are two ways to think about fixed cost. The

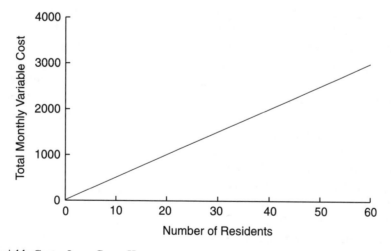

Figure 7–2 Variable Cost—Jones Group Home

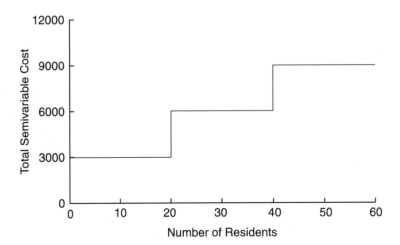

Figure 7–3 Semivariable Cost—Jones Group Home

usual view is the flat line illustrated on the graph in Figure 7–1. That flat line represents total monthly cost for the group home. However, another perception is presented in Figure 7–4. The top view of fixed costs in Figure 7–4 is the usual flat line just discussed. The bottom view is fixed cost per resident. Think about the figure for a moment: the top view is dollars in total for the home for the month, and the bottom view is fixed-cost dollars by number of residents. Note that the line is no longer flat but declines—because this view of cost declines with each additional resident.

We can also think about variable cost in two ways. The usual view of variable cost is the diagonal line rising from the bottom of the graph to the top, as illustrated in Figure 7–2. That steep diagonal line represents monthly cost varying in direct proportion with number of residents in the home. However, another perception is presented in Figure 7–5. The top view of variable costs in Figure 7–5 represents total monthly variable cost and is the usual diagonal line just discussed. The bottom view is variable cost per resident. Think about this figure for a moment: the top view is dollars in total for the home for the month, and the bottom

view is variable-cost dollars by number of residents. Note that the line is no longer diagonal but is now flat—because this view of variable cost stays the same proportionately for each resident. A good way to think about Figures 7–4 and 7–5 is to realize that they are close to being mirror images of each other.

Semifixed costs are sometimes used in health care organizations, especially in regard to staffing. Semifixed costs are the reverse of semivariable costs: that is, they stay fixed for a time as activity levels (or volume) of operations change, but then they will rise; then they will plateau; then they will rise. Thus, semifixed costs can exhibit a step pattern similar to that of variable costs.[2] However, the semifixed cost "steps" tend to be longer between rises in cost. In summary, both semifixed and semivariable costs have mixed elements of fixed and variable costs. Thus, both semivariable and semifixed costs are called *mixed costs*.

EXAMPLES OF VARIABLE AND FIXED COSTS

Studying examples of expenses that are designated as variable and fixed helps to un-

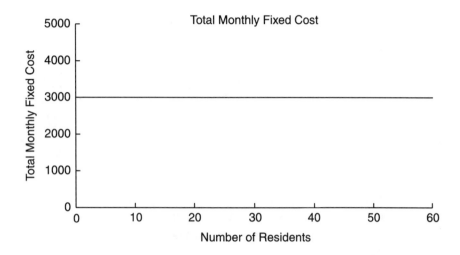

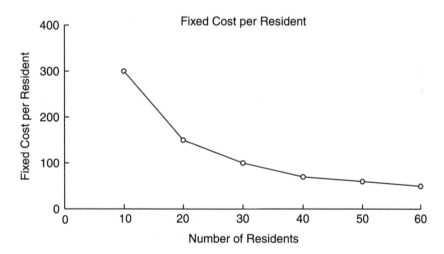

Figure 7–4 Two Views of Fixed Costs

derstand the differences between them. It should also be mentioned that some expenses can be variable to one organization and fixed to another because they are handled differently by the two organizations. Operating room fixed and variable costs are illustrated in Table 7–1. Thirty-two expense accounts are listed in this table: 11 are variable, 20 are designated as fixed by this hospital, and 1, equipment depreciation, is listed separately.[1]

(The separate listing is because of the way this hospital's accounting system handles equipment depreciation.)

Another example of semivariable and fixed staffing is presented in Table 7–2. The costs are expressed as full-time equivalent staff, or FTEs. Each line-item FTE will be multiplied times the appropriate wage or salary to obtain the semivariable and fixed costs for the operating room. (The further use of

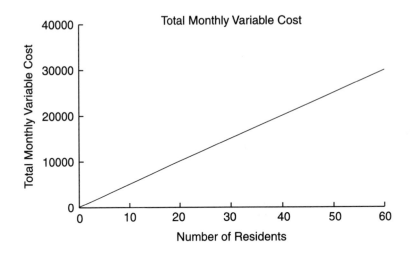

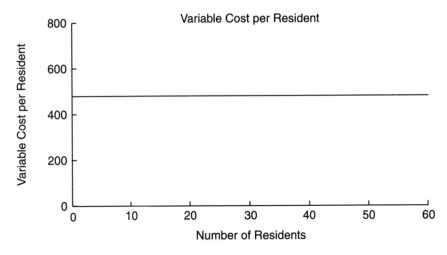

Figure 7–5 Two Views of Variable Costs

FTEs for staffing purposes is fully discussed in the next chapter.) Note that the supervisor position is fixed, which indicates that this is the minimum staffing that can be allowed. The single aide/orderly and the clerical position are also indicated as fixed. All the other positions—technicians, RNs, and LPNs—are listed as semivariable, which indicates that they are probably used in the semivariable step pattern that has been previously discussed in this chapter. This table is a good example of how to show clearly which costs will be designated as semivariable and which costs will be designated as fixed.

Another example illustrates the behavior of a single variable cost in a doctor's office. In Table 7–3, we see an array of costs for the procedure code 99214 office visit type. Nine costs are listed. The first cost is variable and shall be discussed momentarily. The other eight costs are all shown at the same level for a 99214 office visit: supplies, for example, is

Table 7–1 Operating Room Fixed and Variable Costs

Account	Total	Variable	Fixed	Equipment
Social Security	$60,517	$60,517	$	$
Pension	20,675	20,675		
Health Insurance	8,422	8,422		
Child Care	4,564	4,564		
Patient Accounting	155,356	155,356		
Admitting	110,254	110,254		
Medical Records	91,718	91,718		
Dietary	27,526	27,526		
Medical Waste	2,377	2,377		
Sterile Procedures	78,720	78,720		
Laundry	40,693	40,693		
Depreciation—Equipment	87,378			87,378
Depreciation—Building	41,377		41,377	
Amortization—Interest	(5,819)		(5,819)	
Insurance	4,216		4,216	
Administration	57,966		57,966	
Medical Staff	1,722		1,722	
Community Relations	49,813		49,813	
Materials Management	64,573		64,573	
Human Resources	31,066		31,066	
Nursing Administration	82,471		82,471	
Data Processing	17,815		17,815	
Fiscal	17,700		17,700	
Telephone	2,839		2,839	
Utilities	26,406		26,406	
Plant	77,597		77,597	
Environmental Services	32,874		32,874	
Safety	2,016		2,016	
Quality Management	10,016		10,016	
Medical Staff	9,444		9,444	
Continuous Quality Improvement	4,895		4,895	
EE Health	569		569	
Total Allocated	$1,217,756	$600,822	$529,556	$87,378

Source: Adapted from J.J. Baker, *Activity-Based Costing and Activity-Based Management for Health Care*, p. 191, © 1998, Aspen Publishers, Inc.

the same amount in all four columns. The single figure that varies is the top line, which is "report," meaning lab reports. This cost directly varies with the proportion of activity or volume, as variable cost has been defined. Here we see a variable cost at work: the first column on the left has no lab report, and the cost is zero; the second column has one lab report, and the cost is $3.82; the third column has two lab reports, and the cost is $7.64; and the fourth column has three lab reports, and the cost is $11.46. Note also that the total cost rises by the same proportionate increase as the increase in the first line.

Table 7–2 Operating Room Semivariable and Fixed Staffing

Job Positions	Total No. of FTEs	Semivariable	Fixed
Supervisor	2.2		2.2
Techs	3.0	3.0	
RNs	7.7	7.7	
LPNs	1.2	1.2	
Aides, orderlies	1.0		1.0
Clerical	1.2		1.2
Totals	16.3	11.9	4.4

ANALYZING MIXED COSTS

It is important for planning purposes for the manager to know how to deal with mixed costs because they occur so often. For example, telephone, maintenance, repairs, and utilities are all actually mixed costs. The fixed portion of the cost is that portion representing having the service (such as telephone) ready to use, and the variable portion of the cost represents a portion of the charge for actual consumption of the service. We will briefly discuss two very simple methods of analyzing mixed costs. Then we will ex-

amine the high-low method and the scatter graph method.

Predominant Characteristics and Step Methods

Both the predominant characteristics and the step method of analyzing mixed costs are quite simple. In the predominant characteristic method, the manager judges whether the cost is more fixed or more variable and acts on that judgment. In the step method, the manager examines the "steps" in the step pattern of mixed cost and decides whether the cost appears to be more fixed or more variable. Both methods are subjective.

High-Low Method

As the term implies, the high-low method of analyzing mixed costs requires that the cost be examined at its high level and at its low level. To compute the amount of variable cost involved, the difference in cost between high and low levels is obtained and is divided by the amount of change in the activity (or volume). Two examples will be examined.

The first example is for an employee cafeteria. Table 7–4 contains the basic data re-

Table 7–3 Office Visit with Variable Cost of Tests

Service Code	99214 No Test	99214 1 Test	99214 2 Tests	99214 3 Tests
Report of lab tests	**0.00**	**3.82**	**7.64**	**11.46**
Fixed overhead	$31.00	$31.00	$31.00	$31.00
Physician	11.36	11.36	11.36	11.36
Medical assistant	1.43	1.43	1.43	1.43
Bill	0.45	0.45	0.45	0.45
Checkout	1.00	1.00	1.00	1.00
Receptionist	1.28	1.28	1.28	1.28
Collection	0.91	0.91	0.91	0.91
Supplies	0.31	0.31	0.31	0.31
Total visit cost	$47.74	$51.56	$55.38	$59.20

Table 7–4 Employee Cafeteria Number of Meals and Cost by Month

Month	No. of Meals	Employee Cafeteria Cost ($)
July	40,000	164,000
August	43,000	167,000
September	45,000	165,000
October	41,000	162,000
November	37,000	164,000
December	33,000	146,000
January	28,000	123,000
February	22,000	91,800
March	20,000	95,000
April	25,000	106,800
May	30,000	130,200
June	35,000	153,000

quired for the high-low computation. With the formula described in the preceding paragraph, the following steps are performed:

1. Find the highest volume of 45,000 meals at a cost of $165,000 in September (see Table 7–4) and the lowest volume of 20,000 meals at a cost of $95,000 in March.
2. Compute the variable rate per meal as

	No. of Meals	Employee Cafeteria Cost
Highest volume	45,000	$165,000
Lowest volume	20,000	95,000
Difference	25,000	70,000

3. Divide the difference in cost ($70,000) by the difference in number of meals (25,000) to arrive at the variable cost rate:

$70,000 divided by 25,000 meals = $2.80 per meal

4. Compute the fixed overhead rate as follows:

a. At the highest level:

Total cost	$165,000
Less: variable portion	
[45,000 meals × $2.80 @]	(126,000)
Fixed portion of cost	$39,000

b. At the lowest level:

Total cost	$95,000
Less: variable portion	
[20,000 meals × $2.80 @]	(56,000)
Fixed portion of cost	$39,000

c. Proof totals: $39,000 fixed portion at both levels

The manager should recognize that large or small dollar amounts can be adapted to this method. A second example concerns drug samples and their cost. In this example, a supervisor of marketing is concerned about the number of drug samples used by the various members of the marketing staff. She uses the high-low method to determine the portion of fixed cost. Table 7–5 contains the basic data required for the high-low computation. Using the formula previously described, the following steps are performed:

1. Find the highest volume of 1,000 samples at a cost of $5,000 (see Table 7–5) and the lowest volume of 750 samples at a cost of $4,200.

Table 7–5 Number of Drug Samples and Cost for November

Rep.	No. of Samples	Cost
J. Smith	1,000	5,000
A. Jones	900	4,300
B. Baker	850	4,600
G. Black	975	4,500
T. Potter	875	4,750
D. Conner	750	4,200

2. Compute the variable rate per sample as:

	No. of Samples	Cost
Highest volume	1,000	$5,000
Lowest volume	750	4,200
Difference	250	$800

3. Divide the difference in cost ($800) by the difference in number of samples (250) to arrive at the variable cost rate:

$800 divided by 250 samples = $3.20 per sample

4. Compute the fixed overhead rate as follows:

   a. At the highest level:

Total cost	$5,000
Less: variable portion	
[1,000 samples × $3.20 @]	(3,200)
Fixed portion of cost	$1,800

   b. At the lowest level:

Total cost	$4,200
Less: variable portion	
[750 samples × $3.20 @]	(2,400)
Fixed portion of cost	$1,800

   c. Proof totals: $1,800 fixed portion at both levels

The high-low method is an approximation that is based on the relationship between the highest and the lowest levels, and the computation assumes a straight-line relationship. The advantage of this method is its convenience in the computation method.

CONTRIBUTION MARGIN, CVP AND PV RATIOS

The manager should know how to analyze the relationship of cost, volume, and profit. This important information assists the manager in properly understanding and controlling operations. The first step in such analysis is the computation of the contribution margin.

Contribution Margin

The contribution margin is calculated in this way:

		% of Revenue
Revenues (net)	$500,000	100%
Less: variable cost	(350,000)	70%
Contribution margin	$150,000	30%
Less: fixed cost	(120,000)	
Operating income	$30,000	

The contribution margin of $150,000 or 30 percent in this example represents variable cost deducted from net revenues. The answer represents the contribution margin, so called because it contributes to fixed costs and to profits.

The importance of dividing costs into fixed and variable becomes apparent now, for a contribution margin computation demands either fixed or variable cost classifications; no mixed costs are recognized in this calculation.

Cost-Volume-Profit (CVP) Ratio or Breakeven

The breakeven point is the point when the contribution margin (i.e., net revenues less variable costs) equals the fixed costs. When operations exceeds this breakeven point, an excess of revenues over expenses (income) is realized. But if operations does not reach the breakeven point, there will be an excess of expenses over revenues, and a loss will be realized.

The manager must recognize there are two ways of expressing the breakeven point: either by an amount per unit or as a percentage of net revenues. If the contribution margin is expressed as a percentage of net revenues, it is often called the profit-volume (PV) ratio. A PV ratio example follows this cost-volume-profit (CVP) computation.

The CVP example is given in Figure 7–6. The data points for the chart come from the contribution margin as already computed:

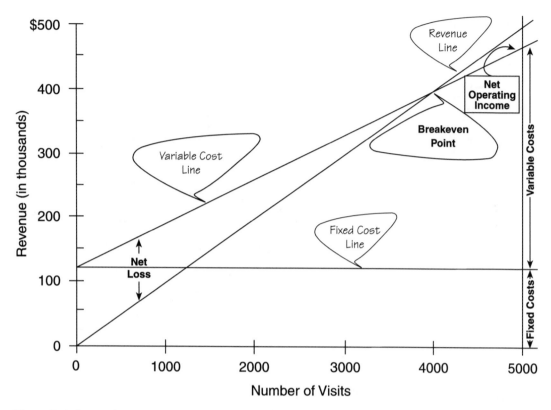

Figure 7–6 Cost-Volume-Profit (CVP) Chart for a Wellness Clinic. Courtesy of Resource Group, Ltd., Dallas, Texas.

		% of Revenue
Revenues (net)	$500,000	100%
Less: variable cost	(350,000)	70%
Contribution margin	$150,000	30%
Less: fixed cost	(120,000)	
Operating income	$30,000	

Three lines were first drawn to create the chart. They were total fixed costs of $120,000, total revenue of $500,000, and variable costs of $350,000. (All three are labeled on the chart.) The breakeven point appears at the point where the total cost line intersects the revenue line. Because this point is indeed the breakeven point, the organization will have no profit and no loss but will break even. The wedge shape to the left of the breakeven point is potential net loss, whereas the more narrow wedge to the right is potential net income (both are labeled on the chart).

CVP charts allow a visual illustration of the relationships that are very effective for the manager.

Profit-Volume (PV) Ratio

Remember that the second method of expressing the breakeven point is as a percentage of net revenues and that if the contribution margin is expressed as a percentage of net revenues, it is called the profit-volume (PV) ratio. Figure 7–7 illustrates the method. The basic data points used for the chart were as follows:

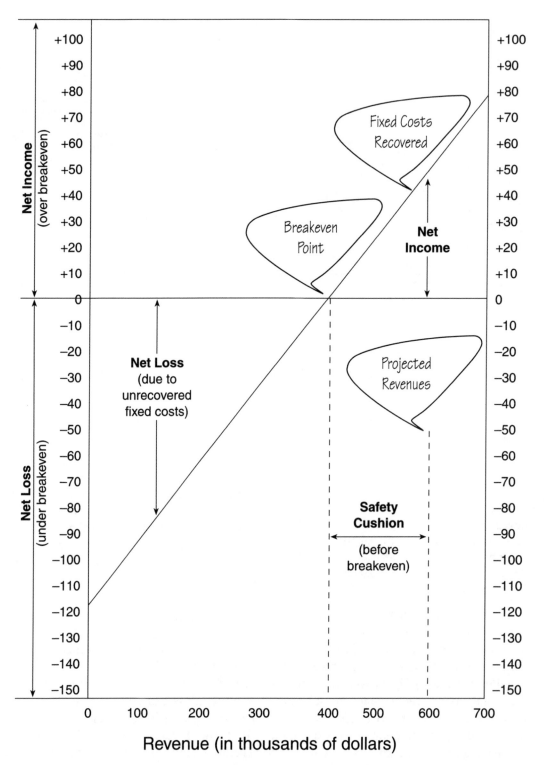

Figure 7–7 Profit-Volume (PV) Chart for a Wellness Clinic. Courtesy of Resource Group, Ltd., Dallas, Texas.

Revenue per visit	$100.00	100%
Less variable cost per visit	(70.00)	70%
Contribution margin per visit	$30.00	30%
Fixed costs per period	$120,000	

$30.00 contribution margin per visit divided by $100 price per visit = 30% PV Ratio

On our chart, the profit pattern is illustrated by a line drawn from the beginning level of fixed costs to be recovered ($120,000 in our case). Another line has been drawn straight across the chart at the breakeven point. When the diagonal line begins at $120,000, its intersection with the breakeven or zero line is at $400,000 in revenue (see left-hand dotted line on chart). We can prove out the $120,000 versus $400,000 relationship as follows. Each dollar of revenue reduces the potential of loss by $0.30 (or 30 percent × $1.00). Fixed costs are fully recovered at a revenue level of $400,000, proved out as $120,000 divided by .30 = $400,000. This can be written as:

$$.30 R = \$120,000$$
$$R = \$400,000 \ [120,000 \ \text{divided by}$$
$$.30 = 400,000].$$

The PV chart is very effective in planning meetings because only two lines are necessary to show the effect of changes in volume. Both PV and CVP are useful when working with the effects of changes in breakeven points and revenue volume assumptions.

Contribution margins are also useful for showing profitability in other ways. An example appears in Figure 7–8, which shows the profitability of various DRGs, using contribution margins as the measure of profitability. Case volume (the number of cases of each DRG) is on the vertical axis of the matrix, and the dollar amount of contribution margin is on the horizontal axis of the matrix.

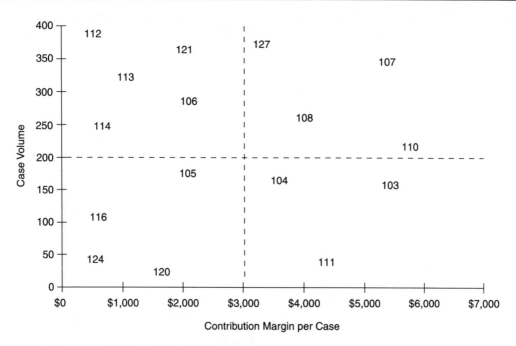

Figure 7–8 Profitability Matrix for Various DRGs, Using Contribution Margins. *Source:* Adapted from S. Upda, Activity-Based Costing for Hospitals, *Health Care Management Review,* Vol. 21, No. 3, p. 85, © 1996, Aspen Publishers, Inc.

Scatter Graph Method

In performing a mixed-cost analysis, the manager is attempting to find the mixed cost's average rate of variability. The scatter graph method is more accurate than the high-low method previously described. It uses a graph to plot all points of data, rather than the highest and lowest figures used by the high-low method. Generally, cost will be on the vertical axis of the graph, and volume will be on the horizontal axis. All points are plotted, each point being placed where cost and volume intersect for that line item. A regression line is then fitted to the plotted points. The regression line basically represents the average—or a line of averages. The average total fixed cost is found at the point where the regression line intersects with the cost axis.

Two examples will be examined. They match the high-low examples previously calculated. Figure 7–9 presents the cafeteria data. The costs for cafeteria meals have been plotted on the graph, and the regression line has been fitted to the plotted data points. The regression line strikes the cost axis at a certain point; that amount represents the fixed cost portion of the mixed cost. The balance (or the total less the fixed cost portion) represents the variable portion.

The second example also matches the high-low example previously calculated. Figure 7–10 presents the drug sample data. The costs for drug samples have been plotted on the graph, and the regression line has been fitted to the plotted data points. The regression line again strikes the cost axis at the point representing the fixed-cost portion of the mixed cost. The balance (the total less the fixed cost portion) represents the variable portion. Further discussions of this method can be found in Exercises and Examples at the back of this book.

The examples presented here have regression lines fitted visually. However, computer programs are available that will place the regression line through statistical analysis as a function of the program. This method is

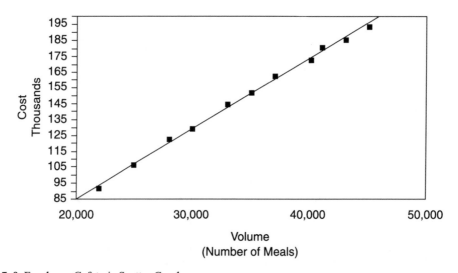

Figure 7–9 Employee Cafeteria Scatter Graph

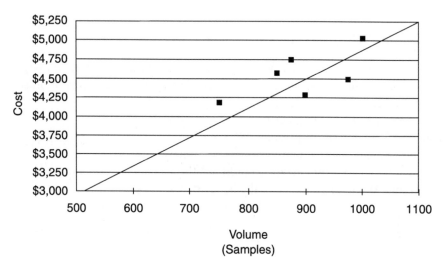

Figure 7–10 Drug Sample Scatter Graph for November

called the least-squares method. *Least squares* means that the sum of the squares of the deviations from plotted points to regression line is smaller than would occur from any other way the line could be fitted to the data: in other words, it is the best fit. This method is, of course, more accurate than fitting the regression line visually.

 INFORMATION CHECKPOINT

What Is Needed?	Revenues, variable cost, and fixed cost for a unit, division, DRG, etc.
Where Is It Found?	In operating reports.
How Is It Used?	Use the multiple-step calculations in this chapter to compute the CPV or the PV ratio; use to plan and control operations.

 KEY TERMS

Breakeven Analysis
Cost-Profit-Volume (CPV)
Contribution margin
Fixed Cost
Mixed Cost
Profit-Volume (PV) Ratio
Semifixed Cost
Semivariable Cost
Variable Cost

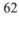

DISCUSSION QUESTIONS

1. Have you seen reports in your workplace that set out the contribution margin?
2. Do you believe that contribution margins can help you manage in your present work? In the future? How?
3. Have you encountered breakeven analysis in your work?
4. If so, how was it used (or presented)?
5. How do you think you would use breakeven analysis?
6. Do you believe your organization could use these analysis tools more often than is now happening? What do you believe the benefits would be?

CHAPTER 8

Staffing: The Manager's Responsibility

PROGRESS NOTES

After completing this chapter, you should be able to

1. Understand the difference between productive time and nonproductive time.
2. Understand computing full-time equivalents (FTEs) to annualize staff positions.
3. Understand computing FTEs to fill a scheduled position.
4. Tie cost to staffing.

STAFFING REQUIREMENTS

In most businesses, a position is filled if the employee works five days a week, generally Monday through Friday. But in health care, many positions must be filled, or covered, all seven days of the week. Furthermore, in most businesses, a position is filled for that day if the employee works an eight-hour day—from 9:00 to 5:00, for example. But in health care, many positions must also be filled, or covered, 24 hours a day. The patients need care on Saturday and Sunday as well as Monday through Friday, and patients need care around the clock, 24 hours a day.

Thus, health care employees work in shifts. The shifts are often eight-hour shifts, because three such shifts times eight hours apiece equals 24-hour coverage. Some facilities have gone to 12-hour shifts. In their case, two 12-hour shifts equals 24-hour coverage. The manager is responsible for seeing that an employee is present and working for each position and for every shift required for that position. Therefore, it is necessary to understand and use the staffing measurement known as the full-time equivalent (FTE). There are two different approaches to computing FTEs: the annualizing method and the scheduled-position method. Full-time equivalent is a measure to express the equivalent of an employee (annualized) or a position (staffed) for the full time required. We will examine both methods in this chapter.

FTEs FOR ANNUALIZING POSITIONS

Why Annualize?

Annualizing is necessary because each employee that is eligible for benefits (such as vacation days) will not be on duty for the full number of hours paid for by the organization. Annualizing thus allows the full cost of the position to be computed through a "burden" approach. In the "burden" approach, the net hours desired are inflated, or burdened, in order to arrive at the gross number of paid hours that will be needed to obtain the desired number of net hours on duty from the employee.

Productive versus Nonproductive Time

Productive time actually equates to the employee's net hours on duty when perform-ing the functions in his or her job description. Nonproductive time is paid-for time when the employee is not on duty: that is, not produc-ing and therefore "nonproductive." Paid-for vacation days, holidays, personal leave days, and/or sick days are all nonproductive time.[1]

Exhibit 8–1 illustrates productive time (net days when on duty) versus nonproductive time (additional days paid for but not

---

Exhibit 8–1 Metropolis Clinic Security Guard Staffing

The Metropolis laboratory area has its own security guard from 8:30 AM to 4:30 PM seven days per week. Bob, the security guard for the clinic area, is a full-time Metropolis employee.
He works as follows:

1. The area assigned to Bob is covered seven days per week for every week of the year.
   Therefore,

Total days in business year	364

2. Bob doesn't work on weekends   (104)
   (2 days per week × 52 weeks = 104 days)

   Bob's paid days total per year amount to   260
   (5 days per week × 52 weeks = 260 days)

3. During the year Bob gets paid for:

Holidays	9	
Sick days	7	
Vacation days	7	
Education days	2	
		(25)

4. Net paid days Bob actually works   235

Jim, a police officer, works part time as a security guard for the Metropolis laboratory area. Jim works on the days when Bob is off, including:

Weekends	104	
Bob's holidays	9	
Bob's sick days	7	
Bob's vacation days	7	
Bob's education days	2	
	129	

5. Paid days Jim works   129

6. Total days lab area security guard position is covered   364

worked). In Exhibit 8–1, Bob, the security guard, is paid for 260 days per year (total paid days) but works for only 235 days per year. The 235 days are productive time, and the remaining 25 days of holiday, sick days, vacation days, and education days are nonproductive time.

FTE for Annualizing Positions Defined

For purposes of annualizing positions, the definition of FTE is as follows: the equivalent of one full-time employee paid for one year, including both productive and nonproductive (vacation, sick, holiday, education, etc.) time. Two employees each working half-time for one year would be the same as one FTE.[2]

Staffing Calculations To Annualize Positions

Exhibit 8–2 contains a two-step process to perform the staffing calculation by the annualizing method. The first step computes the net paid days worked. In this step, the number of paid days per year is first arrived at; then

---

Exhibit 8–2 Basic Calculation for Annualizing Master Staffing Plan

Step 1: Compute Net Paid Days Worked

	RN	LPN	NA
Total Days in Business Year	364	364	364
Less Two Days off per Week	104*	104*	104*
No. of Paid Days per Year	260	260	260
Less Paid Days Not Worked:			
Holidays	9	9	9
Sick Days	7	7	7
Vacation Days	15	15	15
Education Days	3	2	1
Net Paid Days Worked	226	227	228

Step 2: Convert Net Paid Days Worked to a Factor

RN   Total days in business year divided by net paid days worked equals factor 364/226 = 1.6106195

LPN Total days in business year divided by net paid days worked equals factor 364/227 = 1.6035242

NA   Total days in business year divided by net paid days worked equals factor 364/228 = 1.5964912

*Two days off per week equals $52 \times 2 = 104$.

Source: Data from J.J. Baker, *Prospective Payment for Long Term Care,* p. 116, © 1998, Aspen Publishers, Inc. and S.A. Finkler, *Budgeting Concepts for Nurse Managers,* 2nd ed., pp. 174–185, © 1992, W.B. Saunders Company.

paid days not worked are deducted to arrive at net paid days worked. The second step of the staffing calculation converts the net paid days worked to a factor. In the example in Exhibit 8–2, the factor averages out to about 1.6.

This calculation is for a 24-hour around-the-clock staffing schedule. Thus, the 364 in the step 2 formula equates to a 24-hour staffing expectation. Exhibit 8–3 illustrates such a master staffing plan.

NUMBER OF EMPLOYEES REQUIRED TO FILL A POSITION: ANOTHER WAY TO CALCULATE FTEs

Why Calculate by Position?

The calculation of number of FTEs by the schedule position method—in other words, to fill a position—is used in controlling, planning, and decision making. Exhibit 8–4 sets out the schedule and the FTE computation. A summarized explanation of the calculation in Exhibit 8–4 is as follows. One full-time employee (as shown) works 40 hours per week. One eight-hour shift per day times seven days per week equals 56 hours on duty. Therefore, to cover seven days per week or 56 hours requires 1.4

times a 40-hour employee (56 hours divided by 40 hours equals 1.4), or 1.4 FTEs.

Staffing Calculations To Fill Scheduled Positions

The term "staffing" as used here means the assigning of staff to fill scheduled positions. The staffing measure used to compute coverage is also called the FTE. It measures what proportion of one single full-time employee is required to equate the hours required (e.g., full time equivalent) for a particular position. For example, the cast room has to be staffed 24 hours a day seven days a week because it supports the emergency room and therefore has to provide service at any time. In this example, the employees are paid for an eight-hour shift. The three shifts required to fill the position for 24 hours are called the day shift (7:00 AM to 3:00 PM), the evening shift (3:00 PM to 11:00 PM), and the night shift (11:00 PM to 7:00 AM).

One eight-hour shift times five days per week equals a 40-hour work week. One 40-hour work week times 52 weeks equals a person-year of 2,080 hours. Therefore, one person-year of 2,080 hours equals a full-time

---

Exhibit 8–3 Subacute Unit Master Staffing Plan

	Staffing for Eight-Hour Nursing Shifts						
	Shift 1 Day	+	Shift 2 Evening	+	Shift 3 Night	=	24-Hour Staff Total
RN	2		2		1		5
LPN	1		1		1		3
NA	5		4		2		11

Source: Adapted from J.J. Baker, *Prospective Payment for Long Term Care*, p. 116, © 1998, Aspen Publishers, Inc.

Exhibit 8–4 Staffing Requirements Example

Emergency Department Scheduling for Eight-Hour Shifts:					
	Shift 1 Day	Shift 2 Evening	Shift 3 Night	=	24-Hour Scheduling Total
Position: Emergency Room Intake	1	1	1	=	3 8-hour shifts
To Cover Position Seven Days per Week Equals FTEs of:	1.4	1.4	1.4	=	4.2 FTEs

One full-time employee works 40 hours per week. One eight-hour shift per day times seven days per week equals 56 hours on duty. Therefore, to cover seven days per week or 56 hours requires 1.4 times a 40-hour employee (56 hours divided by 40 hours equals 1.4), or 1.4 FTEs.

position filled for one full year. This measure is our baseline.

It takes seven days to fill the day shift cast room position from Monday through Sunday, as required. Seven days is 140 percent of five days (seven divided by five equals 140 percent), or, expressed another way, is 1.4. The FTE for the day shift cast room position is 1.4. If a seven-day schedule is required, the FTE will be 1.4.

This method of computing FTEs uses a basic 40-hour work week (or 37-hour work week, or whatever is the case in the particular institution). The method computes a figure that will be necessary to fill the position for the desired length of time, measuring this figure against the standard basic work week. For example, if the standard work week is 40 hours and a receptionist position is to be filled for just 20 hours per week, then the FTE for

Table 8–1 Calculations To Staff the Operating Room

Job Position	No. of FTEs	No. of Annual Hours Paid at 2,080 Hours*	No. of Annual Hours Paid at 1,950 Hours†
Supervisor	2.2	4,576	4,290
Techs	3.0	6,240	5,850
RNs	7.7	16,016	15,015
LPNs	1.2	2,496	2,340
Aides, orderlies	1.0	2,080	1,950
Clerical	1.2	2,496	2,340
Totals	16.3	33,904	31,785

*40 hours per week × 52 weeks = 2,080.
†37.5 hours per week × 52 weeks = 1,950.

Exhibit 8–5 Example of a Payroll Register

Metropolis Health System
Payroll Register

Week Ended _____ June 10, 2000 _____

Employee No.	Name	Hours Worked			Rate	Base Pay	Overtime Premiums	Gross Earnings	Deductions					Net Pay
		Regular	Overtime	Total					Federal Income Tax	Social Security	Medicare Tax			
1071	J.F. Green	40	2	42	14.00	588.00	14.00	602.00	90.30	37.32	8.73			465.65
1084	C.B. Brown	40		40	14.00	560.00		560.00	84.00	34.72	8.62			432.66
1090	K.D. Grey	40		40	10.00	400.00		400.00	60.00	24.80	6.16			309.04
1092	R.N. Black	40	5	45	10.00	450.00	25.00	475.00	71.25	29.45	6.89			367.41

Courtesy of Resource Group, Ltd., Dallas, Texas.

that position would be 0.5 FTE (20 hours to fill the position divided by a 40-hour standard work week). Table 8–1 illustrates the difference between a standard work year at 40 hours per week and a standard work year at 37.5 hours per week.

TYING COST TO STAFFING

In the case of the annualizing method, the factor of 1.6 already has this organization's vacation, holiday, sick pay, and other nonproductive days accounted for in the formula. (Review Exhibit 8–2 to check out this fact.) Therefore, this factor is multiplied times the base hourly rate (the net rate) paid to compute cost.

In the case of the scheduled-position method, however, the FTE figure of 1.4 will be multiplied times a burdened hourly rate. The burden on the hourly rate reflects the vacation, holiday, sick pay, and other nonproductive days accounted for in the formula. (Review Exhibit 8–4 to see the difference.) The scheduled-position method is often used in the forecasting of new programs and services.

Actual cost is attached to staffing in the books and records through a subsidiary journal and a basic transaction record (both discussed

---

Exhibit 8–6 Example of a Time Record

Metropolis Health System
Time Card

Employee _____ J. F. Green _____ No. _____ 1071 _____

Department _____ 3 _____ Week ending _____ June 10 _____

Day	Regular				Overtime		Hours	
	In	*Out*	*In*	*Out*	*In*	*Out*	*Regular*	*Overtime*
Monday	8:00	12:01	1:02	5:04			8	
Tuesday	7:56	12:00	12:59	5:03	6:00	8:00	8	2
Wednesday	7:57	12:02	12:58	5:00			8	
Thursday	8:00	12:00	1:00	5:01			8	
Friday	7:59	12:01	1:01	5:02			8	
Saturday								
Sunday								
						Total regular hours	40	
						Total overtime		2

Courtesy of Resource Group, Ltd., Dallas, Texas.

Exhibit 8–7 Comparative Hours Staffing Report

Biweekly Comparative Hours Report
For the Payroll Period Ending Sept. 20, 2000

Dept. No. 3421
Emergency Room

PR 2301

June 10, 2000

		Actual Productive					Budget				Variance		
	Job Code	Regular Time (1)	Overtime (2)	Non-Productive (3)	Total Hours (4)	FTEs (5)	Productive (6)	Non-Productive (7)	Total Hours (8)	FTEs (9)	Number Hours (10)	Number FTEs (11)	Percent (12)
Mgr Nursing Service	11075	80	0	0	80	1.0	69.8	10.2	80	1	0	0	0
Supv Charge Nurse	11403	383.2	0.1	79	462.3	5.8	456	64	520	6.5	57.7	0.7	11.1%
Medical Assistant	12007	6.2	0	0	6.2	0.1	0	0	0	0	-6.2	-0.1	100.0%
Staff RN	13401	2010.5	32.8	285.8	2329.1	29.1	2012.8	240.8	2253.6	28.2	-75.5	-0.9	-3.4%
Relief Charge Nurse	13403	81.9	4.3	0	86.2	1.1	0	0	0	0	-86.2	-1.1	100.0%
Orderly/Transporter	15483	203.8	38	20	261.8	3.3	279.8	35.3	315.1	3.9	53.3	0.6	16.9%
ER Tech	22483	244.6	27.5	67.9	340	4.3	336.2	34.5	370.7	4.6	30.7	0.3	8.3%
Secretary	22730	58.1	0	0	58.1	0.7	50.5	5.9	56.4	0.7	-1.7	0.0	-3.0%
Unit Coordinator	22780	555.1	35.6	74.9	665.6	8.3	505.4	53.8	559.2	7	-106.4	-1.3	-19.0%
Preadmission Testing Clerk	22818	0	6.5	0	6.5	0.1	0	0	0	0	-6.5	-0.1	100.0%
Patient Registrar	22873	617.5	78.6	105.7	801.8	10.0	718.2	57.8	776	9.7	-25.8	-0.3	-3.3%
Lead Patient Registrar	22874	0	0	0	0	0.0	73.8	6.2	80	1	80.0	1.0	100.0%
Patient Registrar (weekend)	22876	36.7	0	0	36.7	0.5	0	0	0	0	-36.7	-0.5	100.0%
Overtime	29998	0	0	0	0	0.0	38.5	0	38.5	0.5	38.5	0.5	100.0%
Department Totals		4277.6	223.4	633.3	5134.3	64.3	4541	508.5	5049.5	63.1	-84.8	-1.2	0.0

Courtesy of Resource Group, Ltd., Dallas, Texas.

in a preceding chapter). Exhibit 8–5 illustrates a subsidiary journal in which employee hours worked for a one-week period are recorded. Both regular and overtime hours are noted. The hourly rate, base pay, and overtime premiums are noted, and gross earnings are computed. Deductions are noted and deducted from gross earnings to compute the net pay for each employee in the final column.

Exhibit 8–6 illustrates a time card for one employee for a week-long period. This type of record, whether it is generated by a time clock or an electronic entry, is the original record upon which the payroll process is based. Thus, it is considered a basic transaction record. In this example, time in and time out are recorded daily. The resulting regular and overtime hours are recorded separately for each day worked. Although the appearance of the time card may vary, the essential transaction is the same: this recording of daily time is where the payroll process begins.

Exhibit 8–7 represents an emergency department staffing report. Note that actual productive time is shown in columns 1 and 2, with regular time in column 1 and overtime in column 2. Nonproductive time is shown in column 3, and columns 1, 2, and 3 are totaled to arrive at column 4, labeled "Total [actual] Hours." The final actual figure is the FTE figure in column 5.

The report is biweekly and thus is for a two-week period. The standard work week amounts to 40 hours, so the biweekly standard work period amounts to 80 hours. Note the first line item, which is for the manager of the emergency department nursing service. The actual hours worked in column 4 amount to 80, and the actual FTE figure in column 5 is 1.0. We can tell from this line item that the second method of computing FTEs—the FTE computation to fill scheduled positions—has been used in this case. Columns 7 through 9 report budgeted time and FTEs, and columns 10 through 12 report the variance in actual from budget. The budget and variance portions of this report will be more thoroughly discussed in Chapter 10.

In summary, hours worked and pay rates are essential ingredients of staffing plans, budgets, and forecasts. Appropriate staffing is the responsibility of the manager.

INFORMATION CHECKPOINT

What Is Needed?	The original record of time and the subsidiary journal summary.
Where Is It Found?	The original record can be found at any check-in point; the subsidiary journal summary can be found with a supervisor in charge of staffing for a unit, division, etc.
How Is It Used?	It is reviewed as historical evidence of results achieved. It is also reviewed by managers seeking to perform future staffing in an efficient manner.

KEY TERMS

Full-Time Equivalents (FTEs)
Nonproductive Time
Productive Time
Staffing

DISCUSSION QUESTIONS

1. Are you or your immediate supervisor responsible for staffing?
2. If so, do you use a computerized program?
3. Do you believe a computerized program is better? If so, why?
4. Does your organization report time as "productive" and "nonproductive"?
5. If not, do you believe it should? What do you believe the benefits would be?

CHAPTER 9

Comparative Data and Forecasts

PROGRESS NOTES

After completing this chapter, you should be able to

1. Understand and use common sizing.
2. Understand and use trend analysis.
3. Know what is important to managers about comparative analysis of operating data.
4. Know how assumptions affect forecasting results.

COMPARATIVE DATA

Purpose

Comparative analysis is important to managers because it creates a common ground to make judgments for planning, control, and decision-making purposes.

Common Sizing

The process of common sizing puts information on the same relative basis. Generally, common sizing involves converting dollar amounts to percentages. If, for example, total revenue of $200,000 equals 100 percent, then radiology revenue of $20,000 will equal 10 percent of that total. Converting dollars to percentages allows comparative analysis. In other words, comparing the percentages allows a common basis of comparison. Note that common sizing is sometimes called *vertical analysis* (because the computation of the percentages is vertical).

Although such comparisons on the basis of percentages can and should be performed on your own organization's data, comparisons can also be made between or among various organizations. For example, Table 9–1 shows how common sizing allows comparison of liabilities for three different hospitals. In each case, the total liabilities equal 100 percent. Then the current liabilities of hospital 1, for example, are divided by total liabilities to find the proportionate percentage attributable to that line item (100,000 divided by 500,000 equals 20 percent; 400,000 divided by 500,000 equals 80 percent). When all the percentages have been computed, add them to make sure they add to 100 percent. If you use a computer, computation of these percentages is available as a spreadsheet function.

Another example of comparative analysis is contained in Table 9–2. In this case, general services expenses for three hospitals are compared. Once again, the total expense for each hospital becomes 100 percent, and the relative percentage for each of the four line

Table 9–1 Common Sizing Liability Information

	Same Year for All Three Hospitals					
	Hospital 1		Hospital 2		Hospital 3	
Current liabilities	$100,000	20%	$500,000	25%	$400,000	80%
Long-term debt	400,000	80%	1,500,000	75%	100,000	20%
Total liabilities	$500,000	100%	$2,000,000	100%	$500,000	100%

items is computed ($320,000 divided by $800,000 equals 40 percent and so on). The advantage of comparative analysis is illustrated by the "laundry" line item, where the dollar amounts are $80,000, $300,000, and $90,000 respectively. Yet each of these amounts is 10 percent of the total expense for the particular hospital.

Trend Analysis

The process of trend analysis compares figures over several time periods. Once again, dollar amounts are converted to percentages to obtain a relative basis for purposes of comparison. But now the comparison is across time. If, for example, radiology revenue was $20,000 this period but was only $15,000 for the previous period, the difference between the two is $5,000. The difference of $5,000 equates to a 33 1/3 percent difference because trend analysis is computed

on the earlier of the two years: that is, the base year (thus, 5,000 divided by 15,000 equals 33 1/3 percent). Note that trend analysis is sometimes called *horizontal analysis* (because the computation of the percentage of difference is horizontal).

An example of horizontal analysis is contained in Table 9–3. In this case, the liabilities of hospital 1 for year 1 are compared to the liabilities of hospital 1's year 2. Current liabilities, for example, were $100,000 in year 1 and are $150,000 in year 2, a difference of $50,000. To arrive at a percentage of difference for comparative purposes, the $50,000 difference is divided by the year 1 base figure of $100,000 to compute the relative differential (thus, 50,000 divided by 100,000 is 50 percent).

Another example of comparative analysis is contained in Table 9–4. In this case, general services expenses for two years in hospital 1 are compared. The difference between

Table 9–2 Common Sizing Expense Information

	Same Year for All Three Hospitals					
	Hospital 1		Hospital 2		Hospital 3	
General services expense						
Dietary	$320,000	40%	$1,260,000	42%	$450,000	50%
Maintenance	280,000	35%	990,000	33%	135,000	15%
Laundry	80,000	10%	300,000	10%	90,000	10%
Housekeeping	120,000	15%	450,000	15%	225,000	25%
Total GS expense	$800,000	100%	$3,000,000	100%	$900,000	100%

Table 9–3 Trend Analysis for Liabilities

| | Hospital 1 | | | | | |
	Year 1		Year 2		Difference	
Current liabilities	$100,000	20%	$150,000	25%	$50,000	50%
Long-term debt	400,000	80%	450,000	75%	50,000	12.5%
Total liabilities	$500,000	100%	$600,000	100%	$100,000	–

year 1 and year 2 for each line item is computed in dollars; then the dollar difference figure is divided by the year 1 base figure to obtain a percentage difference for purposes of comparison. Thus, housekeeping expense in year 1 was $120,000 and in year 2 was $180,000, resulting in a difference of $60,000. The difference amounts to 50 percent ($60,000 difference divided by $120,000 year 1 equals 50 percent). Note also in Table 9–4 that two of the four line items have negative differences: that is, year 2 was less than year 1, resulting in a negative figure. Also note that the dollar figure difference is $100,000 when added down (subtract the negative figures from the positive figures; thus, $85,000 plus $60,000 minus $10,000 minus $35,000 equals $100,000). The dollar figure difference is also $100,000 when

added across ($900,000 minus $800,000 equals $100,000).

Analyzing Operating Data

Comparative analysis is an important tool for managers, and it is worth investing the time to become familiar with both horizontal and vertical analysis. Managers will generally analyze their own organization's data most of the time (rather than performing comparisons against other organizations). With that fact in mind, we will examine operating room operating data (no pun intended) that incorporate both common sizing and trend analysis.

Table 9–5 sets out 32 expense items. The expense amount in dollars for each line item is set out for the current year in the left col-

Table 9–4 Trend Analysis for Expenses

| | Hospital 1 | | | | | |
	Year 1		Year 2		Difference	
General services expense						
Dietary	$320,000	40%	$405,000	45%	$85,000	26.5%
Maintenance	280,000	35%	270,000	30%	(10,000)	(3.5)%
Laundry	80,000	10%	45,000	5%	(35,000)	(43.5)%
Housekeeping	120,000	15%	180,000	20%	60,000	50.0%
Total GS expense	$800,000	100%	$900,000	100%	$100,000	–

Table 9–5 Vertical and Horizontal Analysis for the Operating Room

Account	Comparative Expenses					
	12-Month Current Year	%	12-Month Prior Year	%	Annual Increase (Decrease)	% of Change
Social Security	60,517	4.97	68,177	5.70	(7,660)	−12.66
Pension	20,675	1.70	23,473	1.96	(2,798)	−13.53
Health Insurance	8,422	0.69	18,507	1.55	(10,085)	−119.75
Child Care	4,564	0.37	4,334	0.36	230	5.04
Patient Accounting	155,356	12.76	123,254	10.30	32,102	20.66
Admitting	110,254	9.05	101,040	8.45	9,214	8.36
Medical Records	91,718	7.53	94,304	7.88	(2,586)	−2.82
Dietary	27,526	2.26	35,646	2.98	(8,120)	−29.50
Medical Waste	2,377	0.20	3,187	0.27	(810)	−34.08
Sterile Procedures	78,720	6.46	70,725	5.91	7,995	10.16
Laundry	40,693	3.34	40,463	3.38	230	0.57
Depreciation—Equipment	87,378	7.18	61,144	5.11	26,234	30.02
Depreciation—Building	41,377	3.40	45,450	3.80	(4,073)	−9.84
Amortization—Interest	(5,819)	−0.48	1,767	0.15	(7,586)	130.37
Insurance	4,216	0.35	7,836	0.65	(3,620)	−85.86
Administration	57,966	4.76	56,309	4.71	1,657	2.86
Medical Staff	1,722	0.14	5,130	0.43	(3,408)	−197.91
Community Relations	49,813	4.09	40,618	3.39	9,195	18.46
Materials Management	64,573	5.30	72,305	6.04	(7,732)	−11.97
Human Resources	31,066	2.55	13,276	1.11	17,790	57.27
Nursing Administration	82,471	6.77	92,666	7.75	(10,195)	−12.36
Data Processing	17,815	1.46	16,119	1.35	1,696	9.52
Fiscal	17,700	1.45	16,748	1.40	952	5.38
Telephone	2,839	0.23	2,569	0.21	270	9.51
Utilities	26,406	2.17	38,689	3.23	(12,283)	−46.52
Plant	77,597	6.37	84,128	7.03	(6,531)	−8.42
Environmental Services	32,874	2.70	37,354	3.12	(4,480)	−13.63
Safety	2,016	0.17	2,179	0.18	(163)	−8.09
Quality Management	10,016	0.82	8,146	0.68	1,870	18.67
Medical Staff	9,444	0.78	9,391	0.78	53	0.56
Continuous Quality Improvement	4,895	0.40	0	0.00	4,895	100.00
EE Health	569	0.05	1,513	0.13	(944)	−165.91
Total Allocated	1,217,756	100.00	1,196,447	100.00	21,309	1.75
All Other Expenses	1,211,608	—	—	—	—	—
Total Expense	2,429,364	—	—	—	—	—

umn (beginning with $60,517). The expense amount in dollars for each line item is set out for the prior year in the third column of the analysis (beginning with $68,177). The difference in dollars, labeled "Annual Increase (Decrease)," appears in the fifth column of the analysis (beginning with ($7,660)). Vertical analysis has been performed for the current year, and the percentage results appear in the second column (beginning with 4.97%). Vertical analysis has also been performed for the prior year, and those percentage results appear in the fourth column (beginning with 5.70%). Horizontal analysis has been performed on each line item, and those percentage items appear in the far right column (beginning with –12.66%). This table is a good example of the type of operating data reports that managers receive for planning and control purposes.

FORECASTS

Manager's Use of Forecasts

Forecasted data is information used for purposes of planning for the future. Forecasts can be short range (next year), intermediate range (five years from today), or long range (the next decade and beyond). Forecasting, to some degree or another, is often required when producing budgets. (Budgets are the subject of the next chapter.) It is pretty simple today to create "what if" scenarios on the computer. But the important thing for managers to remember is that assumptions directly affect the results of forecasts.

How Assumptions Affect Forecasted Results

Assumptions Determined by Trend Analysis

One of the basic purposes of performing trend analysis is to compare data between or among years and to see the trends. If such trends are found, then it makes sense to take them into account in your forecast. A word of warning, however: the manager must determine if the data used for comparison in the trend analysis are comparable data.

Assumptions Determined by Payer Changes

Trend analysis is retrospective: that is, it is using historical data from a past period. Fore-

casting is prospective: that is, it is projecting into the future. If changes, say, in regulatory requirements for payment are made this year, then that fact has to be taken into account. Mini-Case Study 2 in Chapter 16 addresses this situation.

Assumptions Determined by Utilization Changes

In health care, significant changes in utilization patterns can be occurring that need to be taken into account in the manager's forecast assumptions. The inexorable shift to shorter lengths of stay for hospital inpatients over the last decade is an example of a basic shift in utilization patterns. Mini-Case Study 2 also addresses this situation.

Staffing Forecasts

Staffing forecasts are a very common type of forecast required of managers. There are three particular pitfalls to be recognized in preparing staffing forecasts: noncontrollable expenses, capacity issues, and labor market issues.

Controllable versus Noncontrollable Expenses

The concept of responsibility centers and controllable versus noncontrollable expenses has been discussed earlier in this book. Essentially, controllable costs are subject to a manager's own decision making, whereas noncontrollable costs are outside that manager's power. It is extremely difficult to make staffing forecasts with any degree of accuracy if noncontrollable expenses are included in the manager's forecast. The organization's structure must be recognized and taken into account when setting up assumptions for staffing forecasts. Shared services across lines of authority are workable in

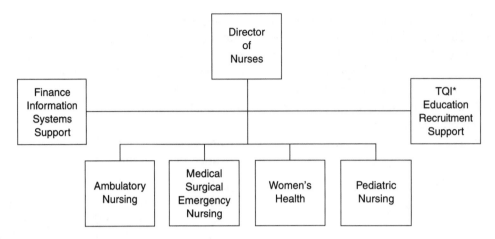

*TQI, total quality improvement.

Figure 9–1 Primary Nursing Staff Classification by Line of Authority. Courtesy of Resource Group, Ltd., Dallas, Texas.

---

theory but often do not work in actuality. Figure 9–1 gives an example of the essential "business units" under the supervision of a director of nurses. Note the responsibility centers and the support centers on this organization chart.

Capacity Issues in Staffing Forecasts

Capacity is a tricky assumption to make in staffing forecasts. In some programs, particularly those in a start-up phase, overcapacity (too much staff available for the amount of work required) is a problem. In some other organizations, undercapacity (a chronic lack of adequate staff) is the problem. Forecasting assumptions, in the best of all worlds, take these difficulties into account. Mini-Case Study 3 in Chapter 18 deals with this problem of staffing in the context of a Women, Infants, and Children (WIC) program.[1]

Labor Market Issues in Staffing Forecasts

The mention of a chronic lack of adequate staff in the preceding paragraph leads us to the problem of the labor market. Certain parts of the country have a continual shortage of certain qualified professional health care staff. Yet other parts of the country can have an overabundance during that same period. The status of the local labor market has a direct impact on staffing forecasts. The impact is in dollars: when there are plenty of staff available, the hourly rate to attract staff goes down, but when there is a shortage of available qualified staff, the hourly rate has to go up. Strange as it may seem, this elemental economic fact is sometimes not taken into account in forecasting assumptions. In summary, the ultimate accuracy of a forecast rests on the strength of its assumptions.

INFORMATION CHECKPOINT

What Is Needed?	An example of a staffing forecast created in your organization.
Where Is It Found?	In the files of the supervisor who is responsible for staffing.
How Is It Used?	Use the example to learn the nature of the assumptions that were used and the setup of the forecast itself.

 KEY TERMS

Common Sizing
Controllable Expenses
Forecasts
Horizontal Analysis
Noncontrollable Expenses
Trend Analysis
Vertical Analysis

 DISCUSSION QUESTIONS

1. Do any of the reports you receive in the course of your work use common sizing? If so, how is it used in your managerial reports?
2. Do any of the reports you work with use trend analysis? If so, how is trend analysis used in your reports?
3. Do you believe there is a better way to present the data for managers in your workplace?
4. Are you or your immediate supervisor involved with staffing decisions? If so, are you aware of how staffing forecasts are done in your organization? Describe an example.

CHAPTER 10

Budgeting and Variance Analysis

PROGRESS NOTES

After completing this chapter, you should be able to

1. Understand the difference between static and flexible budgets.
2. Effectively review a budget.
3. Understand how to build a budget.
4. Perform budget variance analysis.

BUDGETS

A budget is an organizationwide instrument. The organization's objectives define the specific activities to be performed, how they will be assembled, and the particular levels of operation, whereas the organization's performance standards or norms set out the anticipated levels of individual performance. The budget is the instrument through which activities are quantified in financial terms.

A health care standard view of budgeting is illustrated by the American Hospital Association's (AHA's) objectives for the budgeting process:

1. To provide a written expression, in quantitative terms, of a hospital's policies and plans

2. To provide a basis for the evaluation of financial performance in accordance with a hospital's policies and plans
3. To provide a useful tool for the control of costs
4. To create cost awareness throughout the organization[1]

Types of Budgets

Static Budget

A static budget is essentially based on a single level of operations. Once a static budget has been approved and finalized, that single level of operations (volume) is never adjusted. Budgets are measured by how they differ from actual results. Thus, a variance is the difference between an actual result and a budgeted amount when the budgeted amount is a financial variable reported by the accounting system. The variance may or may not be a standard amount, and it may or may not be a benchmark amount.[2]

The computation of a static budget variance only requires one calculation, as follows:

$$\text{Actual Results} - \text{Static Budget Amount} = \text{Static Budget Variance}$$

The basic thing to understand is that static budgeted expense amounts never change when volume actually changes during the year. In the case of health care, we can use patient days as an example of level of volume, or output. Assume that the budget anticipated 400,000 patient days this year (patient days equating to output of service delivery; thus 400,000 output units). Further assume that the revenue was budgeted for the expected 400,000 patient days and that the expenses were also budgeted at an appropriate level for the expected 400,000 patient days. Now assume that only 360,000, or 90 percent, of the patient days are going to actually be achieved for the year. The budgeted revenues and expenses still reflect the original expectation of 400,000 patient days. This example is a static budget; it is geared toward only one level of activity, and the original level of activity remains constant or static.

Flexible Budget

A flexible budget is one that is created using budgeted revenue and/or budgeted cost amounts. A flexible budget is adjusted, or flexed, to the actual level of output achieved (or perhaps expected to be achieved) during the budget period.[3] A flexible budget thus looks toward a range of activity or volume (versus only one level in the static budget).

Flexible budgets became important to health care when diagnosis-related groups (DRGs) were established in hospitals in the 1980s. The development of a flexible budget requires more time and effort than does the development of a static budget. If the organization is budgeting with workload standards, for example, the static budget projects expenses at a single normative level of workload activity, whereas the flexible budget projects expenses at various levels of workload activity.[4]

The concept of the flexible budget addresses workloads, control, and planning.

The budget checklists contained in Appendix A are especially applicable to the flexible budget approach.

Reviewing a Budget

The manager needs to know how to effectively review a budget. To do so, the manager needs to understand how the budget report format is constructed. In general, the usual operating expense budget that is under review will have a column for actual expenditures, a column for budgeted expenditures, and a column for the difference between the two. Usually, the actual expense column and the budget column will both have a vertical analysis of percentages (as discussed in the preceding chapter). Each difference line item will have a horizontal analysis (also discussed in the preceding chapter) that measures the amount of the difference against the budget. Table 10–1 illustrates the operating expense budget configuration just described. Notice that the "Difference" column has both positive and negative numbers in it (the negative numbers being set off with parentheses). Thus, the positive numbers indicate budget overage, such as the dietary line, which had an actual expense of $405,000 against a budget figure of $400,000, resulting in a $5,000 difference. The next line is maintenance. This department did not exceed its budget, so the difference is in parentheses; the maintenance budget amounted to $290,000, and actual expenses were only $270,000, so the $20,000 difference is in parentheses. In this case, parentheses are good (under budget) and no parentheses is bad (over budget).

Another computation the manager needs to know is how to annualize partial-year expenses. Table 10–2 sets out the actual 10-month expenses for the operating room. But these expenses are going to be compared

Table 10–1 Comparative Analysis of Budget versus Actual

	Hospital 1					
	Year 2 Actual		Year 2 Budget		Difference	
	$$	%	$$	%	$$	%
General services expense						
Dietary	$405,000	45	$400,000	46	$5,000	12.5
Maintenance	270,000	30	290,000	33	(20,000)	(6.9)
Laundry	45,000	5	50,000	6	(5,000)	(10.0)
Housekeeping	180,000	20	130,000	15	50,000	38.5
General Service expense	$900,000	100	$870,000	100	$30,000	3.5

against a 12-month budget. What to do? The actual 10-month expenses are converted, or annualized, to a 12-month basis, as shown in the second column of Table 10–2. These computations were performed on a computer spreadsheet; however, the calculation is as follows. Using the first line as an example, $50,431 is 10 months' worth of expenses; therefore, one month's expense is one tenth of $50,431 or $5,043. To annualize for 12 months' worth of expenses, the 10-month total of $50,431 is increased by two more months at $5,043 apiece (50,431 plus 5,043 plus 5,043 equals 60,517, the annualized figure).

Although we have used examples illustrating operating expenses, budgets can, of course, also include revenue. Whether the manager's budget will include revenue (or volume) will generally depend on whether the unit is a responsibility center (discussed in a previous chapter).

A checklist for reviewing a budget appears as Exhibit 10–1. The items are self-explanatory.

Building a Budget

Building a budget means making a series of assumptions. The budget process should begin with a review of strategy and objectives. Forecasting workload is a critical part of building a budget; the workload should tie into expected volume for the new budget period. Good information is necessary to forecast workload. For example, Table 10–3 presents total nursing hours by unit. But there is not enough detail in this report to use because it does not indicate, among other things, hours by type of staff and/or staff level. Sufficient information at the proper level of detail is essential in creating a budget.

Another critical assumption in building a budget is whether special projects are going to use resources during the new budget period. Still another factor to consider is whether operations are going to be placed under some type of unusual or inconvenient circumstances during the new budget period. A good example would be renovation of the work area. Exhibit 10–2 sets out a series of questions and steps to undertake when commencing to build a budget.

To build a flexible budget that looks toward a range of volume, or activity, instead of a single static amount, one must first determine the relevant range of volume, or activity. Thus, the outer limits of fluctuations are determined by defining the relevant range. Next, one must analyze the patterns of the costs expected to occur during the budget period. Third, one must separate the costs by behavior (fixed or variable). Finally, one can prepare the flexible bud-

Table 10–2 Annualizing Operating Room Partial-Year Expenses

	Expenses	
	---	---
Account	Actual 10 Month	Annualized 12 Month
Social Security	50,431	60,517
Pension	17,229	20,675
Health Insurance	7,018	8,422
Child Care	3,803	4,564
Patient Accounting	129,463	155,356
Admitting	91,878	110,254
Medical Records	76,432	91,718
Dietary	22,938	27,526
Medical Waste	1,981	2,377
Sterile Procedures	65,600	78,720
Laundry	33,911	40,693
Depreciation—Equipment	72,815	87,378
Depreciation—Building	34,481	41,377
Amortization—Interest	(4,849)	(5,819)
Insurance	3,513	4,216
Administration	48,305	57,966
Medical Staff	1,435	1,722
Community Relations	41,511	49,813
Materials Management	53,811	64,573
Human Resources	25,888	31,066
Nursing Administration	68,726	82,471
Data Processing	14,846	17,815
Fiscal	14,750	17,700
Telephone	2,366	2,839
Utilities	22,005	26,406
Plant	64,664	77,597
Environmental Services	27,395	32,874
Safety	1,680	2,016
Quality Management	8,347	10,016
Medical Staff	7,870	9,444
Continuous Quality Improvement	4,079	4,895
EE Health	474	569
Total Allocated	1,014,796	1,217,756
All Other Expenses	1,009,673	1,211,608
Total Expense	2,024,469	2,429,364

Source: Adapted from J.J. Baker, *Activity-Based Costing and Activity-Based Management for Health Care*, p. 190, © 1998, Aspen Publishers, Inc.

get—a budget capable of projecting what costs will be incurred at different levels of volume, or activity.

VARIANCE ANALYSIS

This discussion assumes a flexible budget prepared in accordance with the steps just described. A variance is, basically, the difference between standard and actual prices and quantities. Variance analysis analyzes these differences. Flexible budgeting variance analysis was conceived by industry and subsequently discovered by health care. It provides a method to get more information about the composition of departmental expenses. The method subdivides total variance into three types:

1. *Volume variance.* The volume variance is the portion of the overall variance

Exhibit 10–1 Checklist for Reviewing a Budget

1. Is this budget static (not adjusted for volume) or flexible (adjusted for volume during the year)?
2. Are the figures designated as fixed or variable?
3. Is the budget for a defined unit of authority?
4. Are the line items within the budget all expenses (and revenues, if applicable) that are controllable by the manager?
5. Is the format of the budget comparable with that of previous periods so that several reports over time can be compared if so desired?
6. Are actual and budget for the same period?
7. Are the figures annualized?
8. Test one line-item calculation. Is the math for the dollar difference computed correctly? Is the percentage properly computed based on a percentage of the budget figure?

Table 10–3 Nursing Hours Report

Unit		Nursing Hours	
No.	Description	Regular	Overtime
620	S-MED-SURG DIV 5	72,509	6,042
630	N-MED-SURG DIV B	40,248	3,354
640	N-MED SURG DIV D	42,182	3,515
645	N-INTENSIVE CARE UNIT	55,952	4,663
655	S-INTENSIVE CARE UNIT	52,000	4,333
660	S-SURG. ICU	21,840	1,820
665	S-STEPDOWN	52,208	4,351

caused by a difference between the expected workload and the actual workload and is calculated as the difference between the total budgeted cost based on a predetermined, expected workload level and the amount that would have been budgeted had the actual workload been known in advance.[5]

Exhibit 10–2 Checklist for Building a Budget

1. What is the proposed volume for the new budget period?
2. What is the appropriate inflow (revenues) and outflow (cost of services delivered) relationship?
3. What will the appropriate dollar cost be?
   (Note: this question requires a series of assumptions about the nature of the operation for the new budget period.)
   3a. Forecast service-related workload.
   3b. Forecast non–service-related workload.
   3c. Forecast special project workload if applicable.
   3d. Coordinate assumptions for proportionate share of interdepartmental projects.
4. Will additional resources be available?
5. Will this budget accomplish the appropriate managerial objectives for the organization?

2. *Quantity (or use) variance.* The quantity variance is also known as the *use variance* or the *efficiency variance*. It is the portion of the overall variance that is caused by a difference between the budgeted and actual quantity of input needed per unit of output and is calculated as the difference between the actual quantity of inputs used per unit of output multiplied by the actual output level and the budgeted unit price.
3. *Price (or spending) variance.* The price variance is also known as the *spending* or *rate variance*. This variance is the portion of the overall variance caused by a difference between the actual and expected price of an input and is calculated as the difference between the actual and budgeted unit price or hourly rate multiplied by the actual quantity of goods or labor consumed per unit of output and by the actual output level.

Variance analysis can be performed as a two- or a three-variance analysis. (There is also a five-variance analysis that is beyond the scope of this discussion.) The two-variance analysis involves the volume variance as compared to budgeted costs (defined as standard hours for actual production). The three-variance analysis involves the three types of variances defined above. Figure 10–1 illustrates these components.

The makeup of the two-variance is compared to the three-variance in Figure 10–2. As is shown, two elements (A and B) remain the same in both methods. The third element (C) is a single amount in the two-variance method but splits into two amounts (C-1 and C-2) in the three-variance method.

Actual computation is illustrated in Figure 10–3 for two-variance analysis and Figure 10–4, for three-variance analysis. The A, B, C, C-1, and C-2 designations are carried for-

```
┌─────────────────────────────────┐  ┌─────────────────────────────────┐
│          Elements of            │  │          Elements of            │
│      Two-Variance Analysis      │  │     Three-Variance Analysis     │
│                                 │  │                                 │
│  1  Volume Variance             │  │  1  Volume Variance             │
│       (Activity Variance)       │  │       (Activity Variance)       │
│                                 │  │                                 │
│  2  Budget Variance             │  │  2  Quantity Variance           │
│                                 │  │       (Use Variance, Efficiency │
│                                 │  │       Variance)                 │
│                                 │  │                                 │
│                                 │  │  3  Price Variance              │
│                                 │  │       (Spending Variance, Rate  │
│                                 │  │       Variance)                 │
│                                 │  │                                 │
└─────────────────────────────────┘  └─────────────────────────────────┘
```

Figure 10–1 Elements of Variance Analysis. Courtesy of Resource Group, Ltd., Dallas, Texas.

ward from Figure 10–2. In Figure 10–3, the two-variance calculation is illustrated, and a proof total computation is supplied at the bottom of the illustration. In Figure 10–4, the three-variance calculation is likewise illustrated and a proof total computation is also supplied at the bottom of the illustration. This set of three illustrations deserve study. If the

```
┌─────────────────────────────────┐  ┌─────────────────────────────────┐
│         Composition of          │  │         Composition of          │
│      Two-Variance Analysis      │  │     Three-Variance Analysis     │
│                                 │  │                                 │
│  A = Actual Cost Incurred       │  │  A   = Actual Cost Incurred     │
│                                 │  │                                 │
│  B = Applied Cost               │  │  B   = Applied Cost             │
│                                 │  │                                 │
│  C = Budgeted Costs             │  │  C-1 = Budgeted Costs           │
│      (Computed as standard hours│  │        (Computed as actual hours│
│      for actual production)     │  │        for actual production)   │
│                                 │  │                                 │
│                                 │  │  C-2 = Budgeted Costs           │
│                                 │  │        (Computed as standard    │
│                                 │  │        hours for actual         │
│                                 │  │        production)              │
│                                 │  │                                 │
└─────────────────────────────────┘  └─────────────────────────────────┘
```

Figure 10–2 Composition of Two- and Three-Variance Analysis. Courtesy of Resource Group, Ltd., Dallas, Texas.

Variance

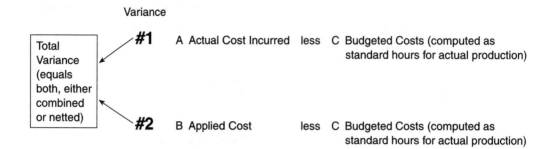

Total
Variance
(equals
both, either
combined
or netted)

#1   A Actual Cost Incurred   less   C Budgeted Costs (computed as
                                            standard hours for actual production)

#2   B Applied Cost   less   C Budgeted Costs (computed as
                                            standard hours for actual production)

Note: To obtain proof total, perform the following calculation:
     A, Actual Cost Incurred, less B, Applied Cost = Total Variance

Figure 10–3 Calculation of Two-Variance Analysis. Courtesy of Resource Group, Ltd., Dallas, Texas.

manager understands the concept presented here, then he or she understands the theory of variance analysis.

Another oddity in variance analysis that contributes to confusion is this. All three variable cost elements—that is, direct materials, direct labor, and variable overhead—can have a price variance and a quantity variance computed. But the variance is not known by the same name in all instances. Exhibit 10–3 sets out the different names. Even though the names differ, the calculation for all three is

Variance

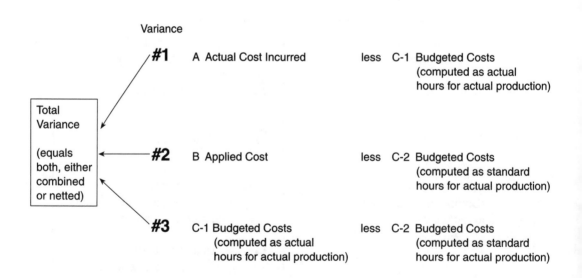

Total
Variance

(equals
both, either
combined
or netted)

#1   A Actual Cost Incurred   less   C-1 Budgeted Costs
                                                (computed as actual
                                                hours for actual production)

#2   B Applied Cost   less   C-2 Budgeted Costs
                                                (computed as standard
                                                hours for actual production)

#3   C-1 Budgeted Costs   less   C-2 Budgeted Costs
         (computed as actual   (computed as standard
         hours for actual production)   hours for actual production)

Note: To obtain proof total, perform the following calculation:
     A, Actual Cost Incurred, less B, Applied Cost = Total Variance

Figure 10–4 Calculation of Three-Variance Analysis. Courtesy of Resource Group, Ltd., Dallas, Texas.

Exhibit 10–3 Different Names for Materials, Labor, and Overhead Variances

Price or Spending Variance = Materials Price Variance	[for direct materials]
Price or Spending Variance = Labor Rate Variance	[for direct labor]
Price or Spending Variance = Overhead Spending Variance	[for variable overhead]

the same. Note, too, that variance analysis is primarily a matter of input-output analysis. The inputs represent actual quantities of direct materials, direct labor, and variable overhead used. The outputs represent the services or products delivered (e.g., produced) for the applicable time period, expressed in terms of standard quantity (in the case of materials) or of standard hours (in the case of labor). In other words, the standard quantity or standard

Exhibit 10–4 St. Joseph Hospital Nursing Center Variance Analysis

Summary Variance Report for Nursing Activity Center

Actual Costs	Flexible Budget (based on actual quantity)	Budgeted Costs
641,331 RVUs × $4.15 per RVU = $2,661,523	641,331 RVUs × $4.50 per RVU = $2,885,989	600,000 RVUs × $4.50 per RVU = $2,700,000

Price Variance	Quantity Variance
= $224,466* (favorable)	= $185,989† (unfavorable)

Assume the following information for the nursing activity center of St. Joseph Hospital for the month of September:

Input Data
Nursing Activity Center
Cost Driver = Number of Relative Value Units (RVUs)

Actual	Budget
Activity Level = 641,331 RVUs	Activity Level = 600,000 RVUs
Overhead Costs = $2,661,523	Overhead Costs = $2,700,000
Actual Cost per RVU = $4.15	Budgeted Cost per RVU = $4.50

*2,885,989 < 2,661,523 > = 224,466
†2,885,989 < 2,700,000 > 185,989.

Source: Adapted from S. Upda, Activity-Based Costing for Hospitals, *Health Care Management Review,* Vol. 21, No. 3, p. 93, © 1996, Aspen Publishers, Inc.

hours equates to what should have been used (the standard) rather than what was actually used. This is an important point to remember.

Example of Variance Analysis

An example of variance analysis in a hospital system is given in Exhibit 10–4. It deals with price or spending variance and quantity or use variance. Note that the price variance is expressed in RVUs. Note also that the quantity variance is broken out into four subtypes—patient, caregiver, environmental, and efficiency variances, all of which are expressed in RVUs. Finally, it is assumed that the budgeted activity level is equal to the standard activity level for purposes of this example.

The flexible budget calculation ($2,885,989) is based on actual quantity. When the $2,885,989 is compared to the actual cost of $2,661,523 for this activity center, a favorable price variance of $224,466 is realized. When the $2,885,989 is compared to the budgeted cost of $2,700,000 for this activity center, an unfavorable quantity variance of ($185,989) is realized.

In closing, when should variances be investigated? Variances will fluctuate within some type of normal range. The trick is to separate normal randomness from those factors requiring correction. The manager would be well advised to calculate the cost-benefit of performing a variance analysis before commencing the analysis.

INFORMATION CHECKPOINT

What Is Needed?   Example of variance analysis performed on a budget.
Where Is It Found?   Possibly with the supervisor responsible for the budget. More likely it will be found in the office of the strategic planner or financial analyst charged with actually performing the analysis.
How Is It Used?   To find where and how variances have occurred during the budget period, in order to manage better in the future.

KEY TERMS

Budget
Flexible Budget
Static Budget
Three-Variance Method
Two-Variance Method
Variance Analysis

DISCUSSION QUESTIONS

1. Do you believe your organization uses a flexible or static budget? Why do you think so?
2. If you reviewed a budget at your workplace, do you think the major increases and decreases could be explained?
3. If so, why? If not, why not?
4. Do you believe variance analysis (or a better variance analysis) would be a good idea at your workplace? If so, why?

CHAPTER 11

The Time Value of Money

<table>
<tr><td rowspan="4">✏️</td></tr>
</table>

PROGRESS NOTES

After completing this chapter, you should be able to

1. Compute an unadjusted rate of return.
2. Understand how to use a present-value table.
3. Compute an internal rate of return.
4. Understand the payback period theory.

PURPOSE

The purpose of these computations is to evaluate the use of money. The manager has many options as to where resources of the organization should be spent.[1] These calculations provide guides to assist in evaluating the alternatives.

UNADJUSTED RATE OF RETURN

The unadjusted rate of return is a relatively unsophisticated return-on-investment method, and the answer is only an estimate, containing no precision. The computation of the unadjusted rate of return is as follows:

$$\frac{\text{average annual net income}}{\text{original investment amount}} = \text{rate of return}$$

OR

$$\frac{\text{average annual net income}}{\text{average investment amount}} = \text{rate of return}$$

The original investment amount is a matter of record. The average investment amount is arrived at by taking the total unrecovered asset cost at the beginning of estimated useful life plus the unrecovered asset cost at the end of estimated useful life and dividing by two. This method has the advantage of accommodating whatever depreciation method has been chosen by the organization. This method is sometimes called the accountant's method because information necessary for the computation is obtained from the financial statements.

PRESENT-VALUE ANALYSIS

The concept of present-value analysis is based on the time value of money. Inherent in this concept is the fact that the value of a dollar today is more than the value of a dollar in the future: thus the "present value" terminology. Furthermore, the further in the future the receipt of your dollar occurs, the less it is worth. Think of a dollar bill dwindling in size more and more as its receipt stretches further and further into the future. This is the concept of present-value analysis.

We learned about compound interest in math class. We learned that

$500 invested at the beginning of year 1
 .05 earns interest (assumed) at a rate of 5%
_____ for one year,
$525 and we have a compound amount at the
      end of year 1 amounting to $525,
 .05 which earns interest (assumed) at the rate
_____ of 5% for another year,
$551 and we have a compound amount at the
      end of year 2 amounting to $551
      (rounded), and so on.

Using this concept, it is possible to restate the present values of $1 to be paid out or received at the end of each of these years. It is possible to use equations, but that is not necessary because we have present value tables (also called "look-up tables," because one can "look-up" the answer). A present value table is included at the end of this chapter in Appendix 11–A. All of the figures on the present value table represent the value of a dollar. The interest rate available on this version of the table is on the horizontal columns and ranges from 1 percent up to 50 percent. The number of years in the period is on the vertical; in this version of the table, the number of years ranges from 1 to 30. To look up a present value, find the column for the proper interest. Then find the line for the proper number of years. Then trace down the interest column and across the number-of-years line item. The point where the two lines meet is the number (or factor) that represents the value of $1 according to your assumptions. For example, find the year 10 by reading down the left-hand column labeled "Year." Then read across that line until you find the

column labeled "10%." The point where the two lines meet is found to be 0.3855. The present value of $1 under these assumptions (10 year/10%) is about 38.5 cents.

Besides using the look-up table, you can also compute this factor on a business calculator. The computation instructions are contained in Appendix B at the back of this book.

Besides using either the look-up table or the business calculator, you can use a function on your computer spreadsheet to produce the factor. The important point is this: no matter which method you use, you should get the same answer.

Now that you have the present value of $1, by whichever method, it is simple to find the present value of any other number. You merely multiply the other number by the factor you found on the table—or in the calculator or the computer. Say, for example, you want to find the present value of $8,000 under the assumption used above (10 years/10%). You simply multiply $8,000 by the factor of 0.3855 you found in the table. The present value of $8,000 is $3,084 (or $8,000 times 0.3855). Note that a compound interest table is also included at the end of this chapter in Appendix 11–B, so you have the tools for computation at your disposal.

INTERNAL RATE OF RETURN

The internal rate of return (IRR) is another return on investment method. It uses a discounted cash flow technique. The internal rate of return is the rate of interest that discounts future net inflows (from the proposed investment) down to the amount invested. The return for a particular investment can therefore be known. The IRR recognizes the elements contained in the previous two methods discussed, but it goes further. It also recognizes the time pattern in which the earnings occur. This means more precision in the computation, because IRR calculates from period to period, whereas the other two methods rely on an average investment.

The IRR computation is not very complicated. The computation requires two assumptions and three steps to compute. Assumption 1: find the initial cost of the investment. Assumption 2: find the estimated annual net cash inflow the investment will generate. Assumption 3: find the useful life of the asset (generally expressed in number of years, known as periods for this computation). Step 1: Divide the initial cost of the investment (assumption #1) by the estimated annual net cash inflow it will generate (assumption #2). The answer is a ratio. Step 2: Now use the look-up table. Find the number of periods (assumption #3). Step 3: Look across the line for the number of periods and find the column that approximates the ratio computed in Step #1. That column contains the interest rate representing the rate of return.

How is IRR used? It can take the rate of return obtained and restate it. The restated figure represents the maximum rate of interest that can be paid for capital over the entire span of the investment without incurring a loss. (You can think of that restated figure as a kind of breakeven point for investment purposes.) The fact that a rate of return can be computed is the benefit of using an IRR method.

PAYBACK PERIOD

The payback period is the length of time required for the cash coming in from an investment to equal the amount of cash originally spent when the investment was acquired. In other words, if we invested $1,000, under a particular set of assumptions, how long would it take to get our $1,000 back? The payback pe-

riod concept is used extensively in evaluating whether to invest in plant and/or equipment. In that case, the question can be restated as: If we invested $1,200,000 in a magnetic resonance imaging machine, under a particular set of assumptions, how long would it take to get the hospital's $1,200,000 back?

The assumptions are key to the computation of the payback period. In the case of equipment, volume of usage is a critical assumption and is sometimes very difficult to predict. Therefore, it is prudent to run more than one payback period computation based on different circumstances. Generally a "best case" and a "worst case" run are made.

The computation itself is simple, although it has multiple steps. The trick is to break it into segments.

For example, Doctor Green is considering the purchase of a machine for his office laboratory. It will cost $300,000. He wants to find the payback period for this piece of equipment. To begin Dr. Green needs to make the following assumptions: Assumption #1: Purchase price of the equipment. Assumption #2: Useful life of the equipment. Assumption #3: Revenue the machine will generate per year. Assumption #4: Direct operating costs associated with earning the revenue. Assumption #5: Depreciation expense per year (computed as purchase price per assumption #1 divided by useful life per assumption #2).

Dr. Green's five assumptions are as follows:

1. Purchase price of equipment = $300,000
2. Useful life of the equipment = 10 years
3. Revenue the machine will generate per year = $10,000 after taxes
4. Direct operating costs associated with earning the revenue = $150,000
5. Depreciation expense per year = $30,000

Now that the assumptions are in place, the payback period computation can be made. It is in three steps, as follows:

Step 1: Find the machine's expected net income after taxes:

Revenue (assumption #3)		$200,000
Less		
Direct operating costs		
(assumption #4)	$150,000	
Depreciation (assumption #5)	30,000	
		180,000
Net income before taxes		$20,000
Less income taxes of 50%		10,000
Net income after taxes		$10,000

Step 2: Find the net annual cash inflow after taxes the machine is expected to generate (in other words, convert the net income to a cash basis):

Net income after taxes	$10,000
Add back depreciation	
(a noncash expenditure)	30,000
Annual net cash inflow after taxes	$40,000

Step 3: Compute the payback period:

$$\frac{\text{investment}}{\text{net annual cash inflow after taxes}} \quad \frac{\$300,000 \text{ machine cost*}}{\$40,000**} = \frac{7.5 \text{ year}}{\text{payback period}}$$

*assumption #1 above
**per step 2 above

The machine will pay back its investment under these assumptions in 7 and one-half years.

Payback period computations are very common when equipment purchases are being evaluated. The evaluation process itself is the final subject we will consider in this chapter.

EVALUATIONS

Evaluating the use of resources in health care organizations is an important task. There are never enough resources to go around, and it is important to use an objective process to evaluate which investments will be made by the organization. A uniform use of a chosen method of evaluating return on investment and/or payback period makes the evaluation process more manageable.

It is important to choose a method that is understood by the managers who will be using it. It is equally important to choose a method that can be readily calculated. If a multiple-page worksheet has to be constructed to set up the assumptions for a modestly priced piece of equipment, the evaluation method is probably too complex. This comment actually touches on the cost-benefit of performing the evaluation.

Sometimes a computer program is chosen that performs a uniform computation of investment returns and payback periods. Such a program is a suitable choice if the managers who use it understand the printouts it produces. Understanding both input and output is key for the managers. In summary, evaluations should be objective, the process should not be too cumbersome, and the responsible managers should understand how the computation was achieved.

 INFORMATION CHECKPOINT

What Is Needed?	Information sufficient to perform these calculations.
Where Is It Found?	In the files of your supervisor; also in the office of the financial analyst; probably also in the strategic planning office.
How Is It Used?	To measure the time value of money.

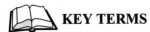 **KEY TERMS**

Internal Rate of Return
Payback Period
Present Value Analysis
Time Value of Money
Unadjusted Rate of Return

 DISCUSSION QUESTIONS

1. Can you compute an unadjusted rate of return now? Would you use it? Why?
2. Are you able to use the present-value look-up table now? Would you prefer a computer to compute it?
3. Have you seen the payback period concept used in your workplace? If not, do you think it ought to be used? What are your reasons?
4. Have you had a chance to participate in an evaluation of an equipment purchase at your workplace? If so, would you have done it differently if you had supervised the evaluation? Why?

Present Value Table
(The Present Value of $1.00)

Year	1%	2%	3%	4%	5%	6%	7%	8%	9%	10%
1	0.9901	0.9804	0.9709	0.9615	0.9524	0.9434	0.9346	0.9259	0.9174	0.9091
2	0.9803	0.9612	0.9426	0.9246	0.9070	0.8900	0.8734	0.8573	0.8417	0.8264
3	0.9706	0.9423	0.9151	0.8890	0.8638	0.8396	0.8163	0.7938	0.7722	0.7513
4	0.9610	0.9238	0.8885	0.8548	0.8227	0.7921	0.7629	0.7350	0.7084	0.6830
5	0.9515	0.9057	0.8626	0.8219	0.7835	0.7473	0.7130	0.6806	0.6499	0.6209
6	0.9420	0.8880	0.8375	0.7903	0.7462	0.7050	0.6663	0.6302	0.5963	0.5645
7	0.9327	0.8706	0.8131	0.7599	0.7107	0.6651	0.6227	0.5835	0.5470	0.5132
8	0.9235	0.8535	0.7894	0.7307	0.6768	0.6274	0.5820	0.5403	0.5019	0.4665
9	0.9143	0.8368	0.7664	0.7026	0.6446	0.5919	0.5439	0.5002	0.4604	0.4241
10	0.9053	0.8203	0.7441	0.6756	0.6139	0.5584	0.5083	0.4632	0.4224	0.3855
11	0.8963	0.8043	0.7224	0.6496	0.5847	0.5268	0.4751	0.4289	0.3875	0.3505
12	0.8874	0.7885	0.7014	0.6246	0.5568'	0.4970	0.4440	0.3971	0.3555	0.3186
13	0.8787	0.7730	0.6810	0.6006	0.5303	0.4688	0.4150	0.3677	0.3262	0.2987
14	0.8700	0.7579	0.6611	0.5775	0.5051	0.4423	0.3878	0.3405	0.2992	0.2633
15	0.8613	0.7430	0.6419	0.5553	0.4810	0.4173	0.3624	0.3152	0.2745	0.2394
16	0.8528	0.7284	0.6232	0.5339	0.4581	0.3936	0.3387	0.2919	0.2519	0.2176
17	0.8444	0.7142	0.6050	0.5134	0.4363	0.3714	0.3166	0.2703	0.2311	0.1978
18	0.8360	0.7002	0.5874	0.4936	0.4155	0.3503	0.2959	0.2502	0.2120	0.1799
19	0.8277	0.6864	0.5703	0.4746	0.3957	0.3305	0.2765	0.2317.	0.1945	0.1635
20	0.8195	0.6730	0.5537	0.4564	0.3769	0.3118	0.2584	0.2145	0.1784	0.1486
21	0.8114	0.6598	0.5375	0.4388	0.3589	0.2942	0.2415	0.1987	0.1637	0.1351
22	0.8034	0.6468	0.5219	0.4220	0.3418	0.2775	0.2257	0.1839	0.1502	0.1228
23	0.7954	0.6342	0.5067	0.4057	0.3256	0.2618	0.2109	0.1703	0.1378	0.1117
24	0.7876	0.6217	0.4919	0.3901	0.3101	0.2470	0.1971	0.1577	0.1264	0.1015
25	0.7798	0.6095	0.4776	0.3751	0.2953	0.2330	0.1842	0.1460	0.1160	0.0923
26	0.7720	0.5976	0.4637	0.3607	0.2812	0.2198	0.1722	0.1352	0.1064	0.0839
27	0.7644	0.5859	0.4502	0.3468	0.2678	0.2074	0.1609	0.1252	0.0976	0.0763
28	0.7568	0.5744	0.4371	0.3335	0.2552	0.1956	0.1504	0.1159	0.0895	0.0693
29	0.7493	0.5631	0.4243	0.3207	0.2429	0.1846	0.1406	0.1073	0.0822	0.0630
30	0.7419	0.5521	0.4120	0.3083	0.2314	0.1741	0.1314	0.0994	0.0754	0.0573

Year	11%	12%	13%	14%	15%	16%	17%	18%	19%	20%
1	0.9009	0.8929	0.8850	0.8772	0.8696	0.8621	0.8547	0.8475	0.8403	0.8333
2	0.8116	0.7972	0.7831	0.7695	0.7561	0.7432	0.7305	0.7182	0.7062	0.6944
3	0.7312	0.7118	0.6913	0.6750	0.6575	0.6407	0.6244	0.6086	0.5934	0.5787
4	0.6587	0.6355	0.6133	0.5921	0.5718	0.5523	0.5337	0.5158	0.4987	0.4823
5	0.5935	0.5674	0.5428	0.5194	0.4972	0.4761	0.4561	0.4371	0.4190	0.4019
6	0.5346	0.5066	0.4803	0.4556	0.4323	0.4104	0.3898	0.3704	0.3521	0.3349
7	0.4817	0.4523	0.4251	0.3996	0.3759	0.3538	0.3332	0.3139	0.2959	0.2791
8	0.4339	0.4039	0.3762	0.3506	0.3269	0.3050	0.2848	0.2660	0.2487	0.2326
9	0.3909	0.3606	0.3329	0.3075	0.2843	0.2630	0.2434	0.2255	0.2090	0.1938
10	0.3522	0.3220	0.2946	0.2697	0.2472	0.2267	0.2080	0.1911	0.1756	0.1615
11	0.3173	0.2875	0.2607	0.2366	0.2149	0.1954	0.1778	0.1619	0.1476	0.1346
12	0.2858	0.2567	0.2307	0.2076	0.1869	0.1685	0.1520	0.1372	0.1240	0.1122
13	0.2575	0.2292	0.2042	0.1821	0.1625	0.1452	0.1299	0.1163	0.1042	0.0935
14	0.2320	0.2046	0.1807	0.1597	0.1413	0.1252	0.1110	0.0985	0.0876	0.0779
15	0.2090	0.1827	0.1599	0.1401	0.1229	0.1079	0.0949	0.0835	0.0736	0.0649
16	0.1883	0.1631	0.1415	0.1229	0.1069	0.0930	0.0811	0.0708	0.0618	0.0541
17	0.1696	0.1456	0.1252	0.1078	0.0929	0.0802	0.0693	0.0600	0.0520	0.0451
18	0.1528	0.1300	0.1108	0.0946	0.0808	0.0691	0.0592	0.0508	0.0437	0.0376
19	0.1377	0.1161	0.0981	0.0829	0.0703	0.0596	0.0506	0.0431	0.0367	0.0313
20	0.1240	0.1037	0.0868	0.0728	0.0611	0.0514	0.0433	0.0365	0.0308	0.0261
21	0.1117	0.0926	0.0768	0.0638	0.0531	0.0443	0.0370	0.0309	0.0259	0.0217
22	0.1007	0.0826	0.0680	0.0560	0.0462	0.0382	0.0316	0.0262	0.0218	0.0181
23	0.0907	0.0738	0.0601	0.0491	0.0402	0.0329	0.0270	0.0222	0.0183	0.0151
24	0.0817	0.0659	0.0532	0.0431	0.0349	0.0284	0.0231	0.0188	0.0154	0.0126
25	0.0736	0.0588	0.0471	0.0378	0.0304	0.0245	0.0197	0.0160	0.0129	0.0105
26	0.0663	0.0525	0.0417	0.0331	0.0264	0.0211	0.0169	0.0135	0.0109	0.0087
27	0.0597	0.0469	0.0369	0.0291	0.0230	0.0182	0.0144	0.0115	0.0091	0.0073
28	0.0538	0.0419	0.0326	0.0255	0.0200	0.0157	0.0123	0.0097	0.0077	0.0061
29	0.0485	0.0374	0.0289	0.0224	0.0174	0.0135	0.0105	0.0082	0.0064	0.0051
30	0.0437	0.0334	0.0256	0.0196	0.0151	0.0116	0.0090	0.0070	0.0054	0.0042

Year	21%	22%	23%	24%	25%	26%	27%	28%	29%	30%
1	0.8264	0.8197	0.8130	0.8065	0.8000	0.7937	0.7874	0.7813	0.7752	0.7692
2	0.6830	0.6719	0.6610	0.6504	0.6400	0.6299	0.6200	0.6104	0.6009	0.5917
3	0.5645	0.5507	0.5374	0.5245	0.5120	0.4999	0.4882	0.4768	0.4658	0.4552
4	0.4665	0.4514	0.4369	0.4230	0.4096	0.3968	0.3844	0.3725	0.3611	0.3501
5	0.3855	0.3700	0.3552	0.3411	0.3277	0.3149	0.3027	0.2910	0.2799	0.2693
6	0.3186	0.3033	0.2888	0.2751	0.2621	0.2499	0.2383	0.2274	0.2170	0.2072
7	0.2633	0.2486	0.2348	0.2218	0.2097	0.1983	0.1877	0.1776	0.1682	0.1594
8	0.2176	0.2038	0.1909	0.1789	0.1678	0.1574	0.1478	0.1388	0.1304	0.1226
9	0.1799	0.1670	0.1552	0.1443	0.1342	0.1249	0.1164	0.1084	0.1011	0.0943
10	0.1486	0.1369	0.1262	0.1164	0.1074	0.0992	0.0916	0.0847	0.0784	0.0725
11	0.1228	0.1122	0.1026	0.0938	0.0859	0.0787	0.0721	0.0662	0.0607	0.0558
12	0.1015	0.0920	0.0834	0.0757	0.0687	0.0625	0.0568	0.0517	0.0471	0.0429
13	0.0839	0.0754	0.0678	0.0610	0.0550	0.0496	0.0447	0.0404	0.0365	0.0330
14	0.0693	0.0618	0.0551	0.0492	0.0440	0.0393	0.0352	0.0316	0.0283	0.0253
15	0.0573	0.0507	0.0448	0.0397	0.0352	0.0312	0.0277	0.0247	0.0219	0.0195
16	0.0474	0.0415	0.0364	0.0320	0.0281	0.0248	0.0218	0.0193	0.0170	0.0150
17	0.0391	0.0340	0.0296	0.0258	0.0225	0.0197	0.0172	0.0150	0.0132	0.0116
18	0.0323	0.0279	0.0241	0.0208	0.0180	0.0156	0.0135	0.0118	0.0102	0.0089
19	0.0267	0.0229	0.0196	0.0168	0.0144	0.0124	0.0107	0.0092	0.0079	0.0068
20	0.0221	0.0187	0.0159	0.0135	0.0115	0.0098	0.0084	0.0072	0.0061	0.0053
21	0.0183	0.0154	0.0129	0.0109	0.0092	0.0078	0.0066	0.0056	0.0048	0.0040
22	0.0151	0.0126	0.0105	0.0088	0.0074	0.0062	0.0052	0.0044	0.0037	0.0031
23	0.0125	0.0103	0.0086	0.0071	0.0059	0.0049	0.0041	0.0034	0.0029	0.0024
24	0.0103	0.0085	0.0070	0.0057	0.0047	0.0039	0.0032	0.0027	0.0022	0.0018
25	0.0085	0.0069	0.0057	0.0046	0.0038	0.0031	0.0025	0.0021	0.0017	0.0014
26	0.0070	0.0057	0.0046	0.0037	0.0030	0.0025	0.0020	0.0016	0.0013	0.0011
27	0.0058	0.0047	0.0037	0.0030	0.0024	0.0019	0.0016	0.0013	0.0010	0.0008
28	0.0048	0.0038	0.0030	0.0024	0.0019	0.0015	0.0012	0.0010	0.0008	0.0006
29	0.0040	0.0031	0.0025	0.0020	0.0015	0.0012	0.0010	0.0008	0.0006	0.0005
30	0.0033	0.0026	0.0020	0.0016	0.0012	0.0010	0.0008	0.0006	0.0005	0.0004

Year	35%	40%	45%	50%
1	0.741	0.714	0.690	0.667
2	0.549	0.510	0.476	0.444
3	0.406	0.364	0.328	0.296
4	0.301	0.260	0.226	0.198
5	0.223	0.186	0.156	0.132
6	0.165	0.133	0.108	0.088
7	0.122	0.095	0.074	0.059
8	0.091	0.068	0.051	0.039
9	0.067	0.048	0.035	0.026
10	0.050	0.035	0.024	0.017
11	0.037	0.025	0.017	0.012
12	0.027	0.018	0.012	0.008
13	0.020	0.013	0.008	0.005
14	0.015	0.009	0.006	0.003
15	0.011	0.006	0.004	0.002
16	0.008	0.005	0.003	0.002
17	0.006	0.003	0.002	0.001
18	0.005	0.002	0.001	0.001
19	0.003	0.002	0.001	
20	0.002	0.001	0.001	
21	0.002	0.001		
22	0.001	0.001		
23	0.001			
24	0.001			
25	0.001			
26				
27				
28				
29				
30				

Compound Interest Table
Compound Amount of $1.00
(The Future Amount of $1.00)

Year	1%	2%	3%	4%	5%	6%	7%	8%	9%	10%
1	1.010	1.020	1.030	1.040	1.050	1.060	1.070	1.080	1.090	1.100
2	1.020	1.040	1.061	1.082	1.102	1.124	1.145	1.166	1.188	1.210
3	1.030	1.061	1.093	1.125	1.156	1.191	1.225	1.260	1.295	1.331
4	1.041	1.082	1.126	1.170	1.216	1.262	1.311	1.360	1.412	1.464
5	1.051	1.104	1.159	1.217	1.276	1.338	1.403	1.469	1.539	1.611
6	1.062	1.120	1.194	1.265	1.340	1.419	1.501	1.587	1.677	1.772
7	1.072	1.149	1.230	1.316	1.407	1.504	1.606	1.714	1.828	1.949
8	1.083	1.172	1.267	1.369	1.477	1.594	1.718	1.851	1.993	2.144
9	1.094	1.195	1.305	1.423	1.551	1.689	1.838	1.999	2.172	2.358
10	1.105	1.219	1.344	1.480	1.629	1.791	1.967	2.159	2.367	2.594
11	1.116	1.243	1.384	1.539	1.710	1.898	2.105	2.332	2.580	2.853
12	1.127	1.268	1.426	1.601	1.796	2.012	2.252	2.518	2.813	3.138
13	1.138	1.294	1.469	1.665	1.886	2.133	2.410	2.720	3.066	3.452
14	1.149	1.319	1.513	1.732	1.980	2.261	2.579	2.937	3.342	3.797
15	1.161	1.346	1.558	1.801	2.079	2.397	2.759	3.172	3.642	4.177
16	1.173	1.373	1.605	1.873	2.183	2.540	2.952	3.426	3.970	4.595
17	1.184	1.400	1.653	1.948	2.292	2.693	3.159	3.700	4.328	5.054
18	1.196	1.428	1.702	2.026	2.407	2.854	3.380	3.996	4.717	5.560
19	1.208	1.457	1.754	2.107	2.527	3.026	3.617	4.316	5.142	6.116
20	1.220	1.486	1.806	2.191	2.653	3.207	3.870	4.661	5.604	6.728
25	1.282	1.641	2.094	2.666	3.386	4.292	5.427	6.848	8.632	10.835
30	1.348	1.811	2.427	3.243	4.322	5.743	7.612	10.063	13.268	17.449

Year	12%	14%	16%	18%	20%	24%	28%	32%	40%	50%
1	1.120	1.140	1.160	1.180	1.200	1.240	1.280	1.320	1.400	1.500
2	1.254	1.300	1.346	1.392	1.440	1.538	1.638	1.742	1.960	2.250
3	1.405	1.482	1.561	1.643	1.728	1.907	2.067	2.300	2.744	3.375
4	1.574	1.689	1.811	1.939	2.074	2.364	2.684	3.036	3.842	5.062
5	1.762	1.925	2.100	2.288	2.488	2.932	3.436	4.007	5.378	7.594
6	1.974	2.195	2.436	2.700	2.986	3.635	4.398	5.290	7.530	11.391
7	2.211	2.502	2.826	3.185	3.583	4.508	5.629	6.983	10.541	17.086
8	2.476	2.853	3.278	3.759	4.300	5.590	7.206	9.217	14.758	25.629
9	2.773	3.252	3.803	4.435	5.160	6.931	9.223	12.166	20.661	38.443
10	3.106	3.707	4.411	5.234	6.192	8.594	11.806	16.060	28.925	57.665
11	3.479	4.226	5.117	6.176	7.430	10.657	15.112	21.199	40.496	86.498
12	3.896	4.818	5.936	7.288	8.916	13.215	19.343	27.983	56.694	129.746
13	4.363	5.492	6.886	8.599	10.699	16.386	24.759	36.937	79.372	194.619
14	4.887	6.261	7.988	10.147	12.839	20.319	31.691	48.757	111.120	291.929
15	5.474	7.138	9.266	11.074	15.407	25.196	40.565	64.350	155.568	437.894
16	6.130	8.137	10.748	14.129	18.488	31.243	51.923	84.954	217.795	656.840
17	6.866	9.276	12.468	16.672	22.186	38.741	66.461	112.140	304.914	985.260
18	7.690	10.575	14.463	19.673	26.623	48.039	85.071	148.020	426.879	1477.900
19	8.613	12.056	16.777	23.214	31.948	59.568	108.890	195.390	597.630	2216.800
20	9.646	13.743	19.461	27.393	38.338	73.864	139.380	257.920	836.683	3325.300
25	17.000	26.462	40.874	62.669	95.396	216.542	478.900	1033.600	4499.880	25251.000
30	29.960	50.950	85.850	143.371	237.376	634.820	1645.500	4142.100	24201.432	191750.000

PART III

Financial Management Tools

CHAPTER 12

Reporting

PROGRESS NOTES

After completing this chapter, you should be able to

1. Review a balance sheet and understand its components.
2. Review a statement of revenue and expense and understand its components.
3. Understand the basic concept of cash flows.
4. Know what a subsidiary report is.

UNDERSTANDING THE MAJOR REPORTS

It is not our intention to convert you into an accountant. Therefore, our discussion of the major financial reports will center on the concept of each report and not on the precise accounting entries that are necessary to make the statement balance. The first concept we will discuss is that of cash versus accrual accounting. In cash basis accounting, a transaction does not enter the books until cash is either received or paid out. In accrual accounting, revenue is recorded when it is earned—not when payment is received—and expenses are recorded when they are incurred—not when they are paid.[1]

Most health care organizations operate on the accrual basis.

There are four basic financial statements. You can think of them as a set. They include the balance sheet, the statement of revenue and expense, the statement of fund balance or net worth, and the statement of cash flows. The four major reports we are about to examine—the financial statements—have been prepared using the accrual method.

BALANCE SHEET

The balance sheet records what an organization owns, what it owes, and, basically, what it is worth (although the terminology uses fund balance rather than worth or equity for nonprofit organizations). The balance sheet balances. That is, the total of what the organization owns—its assets—equals the combined total of what the organization owes and what it is worth—that is, its liabilities and its net worth or its fund balance. This balancing of the elements in the balance sheet can be visualized as:

Assets = Liabilities + Net Worth/Fund Balance

Another characteristic of the balance sheet is that it is stated at a particular point in time. A common analogy is that a balance sheet is like a snapshot: it freezes the figures and reports them as of a certain date.

103

Exhibit 12–1 illustrates these concepts. Note that a single date (not a period of time) is at the top of the statement (this is the snapshot). The clinic balance sheet reflects two years in two columns, with the most current date on the left and the prior period on the right. Total assets for the current left-hand column amount to $963,000. Total liabilities

Exhibit 12–1 Westside Clinic Balance Sheet

Assets	December 31, 20x2		December 31, 20x1	
Currents Assets				
Cash and cash equivalents		$190,000		$145,000
Accounts receivable (net)		250,000		300,000
Inventories		25,000		20,000
Prepaid insurance		5,000		3,000
Total current assets		$470,000		$468,000
Property, Plant, and Equipment				
Land	$100,000		$100,000	
Buildings (net)	0		0	
Equipment (net)	260,000		300,000	
Net property, plant, and equipment		360,000		400,000
Other Assets				
Investments	$133,000		$32,000	
Total other assets		133,000		32,000
Total Assets		$963,000		$900,000
Liabilities and Fund Balance				
Current Liabilities				
Current maturities of long-term debt	$52,000		$48,000	
Accounts payable and accrued expenses	293,000		302,000	
Total current liabilities		$345,000		$350,000
Long-Term Debt	$252,000		$300,000	
Less Current Maturities of Long-Term Debt	(52,000)		(48,000)	
Net Long-Term Debt		200,000		252,000
Total liabilities		$545,000		$602,000
Fund Balances				
Unrestricted fund balance	$418,000		$298,000	
Restricted fund balance	0		0	
Total fund balances		418,000		298,000
Total Liabilities and Fund Balance		$963,000		$900,000

Courtesy of Resource Group, Ltd., Dallas, Texas.

and fund balance also amount to $963,000; the balance sheet balances. Note that the total liabilities amount to $545,000 and the total fund balances amount to $418,000. The total of the two, of course, makes up the $963,000 shown at the bottom of the statement.

Three types of assets are shown: current assets; property, plant, and equipment; and other assets. Current assets are supposed to be convertible into cash within one year—thus "current" assets. Property, plant, and equipment, however, represent long-term assets. Other assets represent noncurrent items.

Two types of liabilities are shown: current liabilities and long-term debt. Current liabilities are those expected to be paid within the next year—thus "current" liabilities. Long-term debt is not due within a year. (In fact, most long-term debt is due over a period of many years.) Notice that the amount of long-term debt that will be due within the next year ($52,000) has been subtracted from the long-term debt amount and has been moved up into the current liabilities section. This treatment is consistent with the concept of "current."

Because our intent is not to make an accountant of you, we will not be discussing generally accepted accounting principles (GAAP) either. Financial accounting and the resulting reports intended for third-party use must be prepared in accordance with GAAP. However, managerial accounting for internal purposes in the organization does not necessarily have to adhere to GAAP. One of the requirements of GAAP is that unrestricted fund balances be separated from restricted fund balances on the statements, so you see two appropriate line items (restricted and unrestricted) in the fund balance section.

STATEMENT OF REVENUE AND EXPENSE

The formula for a very condensed statement of revenue and expense would look like this:

Operating Revenue – Operating Expenses = Operating Income

A statement of revenue and expense covers a period of time (rather than one single date or point in time). The concept is that revenue, or inflow, less expenses, or outflow, results in an excess of revenue over expenses if the year has been good, or perhaps an excess of expenses over revenue (resulting in a loss) if the year has been bad.

Exhibit 12–2 sets out the result of operations for two years, with the most current period in the left columns. If the balance sheet is a snapshot, then the statement of revenue and expenses is a diary, because it is a record of transactions over the period of a year. Notice that operating revenues and operating expenses are set out first, with the result being income from operations of $115,000 ($2,000,000 less $1,885,000). Then other transactions are reported; in this case, interest income of $5,000 under the heading "Nonoperating Gains (Losses)." The total of $120,000 ($115,000 plus $5,000) is reported as an increase in fund balance. This figure carries forward to the next major report, known as the statement of changes in fund balance.

STATEMENT OF CHANGES IN FUND BALANCE/NET WORTH

Remember that our formula for a basic statement of revenue and expense looked like this:

Operating Revenue – Operating Expenses = Operating Income

The excess of revenue over expenses flows back into equity or fund balance through the mechanism of the statement of fund balance/net worth. Exhibit 12–3 shows a balance at the first of the year; then it adds the excess of revenue over expenses (in the amount of

Exhibit 12–2 Westside Clinic Statement of Revenue and Expenses

Revenue	December 31, 20x2	December 31, 20x1
Net patient service revenue	$2,000,000	$1,850,000
Total operating revenue	$2,000,000	$1,850,000
Operating Expenses		
Medical/surgical services	$600,000	$575,000
Therapy services	860,000	806,000
Other professional services	80,000	75,000
Support services	220,000	220,000
General services	65,000	60,000
Depreciation	40,000	40,000
Interest	20,000	24,000
Total operating expenses	1,885,000	1,800,000
Income from Operations	$115,000	$50,000
Nonoperating Gains (Losses)		
Interest income	$5,000	$2,000
Net nonoperating gains	5,000	2,000
Revenue and Gains in Excess of		
Expenses and Losses	$120,000	$52,000
Increase in Unrestricted Fund Balance	$120,000	$52,000

Courtesy of Resource Group, Ltd., Dallas, Texas.

$115,000) plus some interest income (in the amount of $5,000) to arrive at the balance at the end of the year.

If you refer back to the balance sheet, you will see the $418,000 balance at the end of the year appearing on it. So we can think of the balance sheet, the statement of revenue and expenses, and the statement of changes in fund balance/net worth as locked together, with the statement of changes in fund balance being the mechanism that links the other two statements.

But there is one more major report—the statement of cash flows—and we will examine it next.

STATEMENT OF CASH FLOWS

To perceive why a statement of cash flows is necessary, we must first revisit the concept of accrual basis accounting. If cash is not paid or received when revenues and expenses are entered on the books—the usual situation in accrual accounting—what happens? The other side of the entry for revenues is accounts receivable, and the other side of the entry for expenses is accounts payable. These accounts rest on the balance sheet and have not yet been turned into cash. Another characteristic of accrual accounting is the recognition of depreciation. A capital asset—a

Exhibit 12–3 Westside Clinic Statement of Changes in Fund Balance

	For the Year Ending	
Statement of Changes in Fund Balance	December 31, 20x2	December 31, 20x1
Balance First of Year	$298,000	$246,000
Revenue in Excess of Expenses	115,000	50,000
Interest Income	5,000	2,000
Balance End of Year	$418,000	$298,000

Courtesy of Resource Group, Ltd., Dallas, Texas.

piece of equipment, for example—is purchased for $20,000. It has a usable life of five years. So depreciation expense is recognized in each of the five years until the $20,000 is used up, or depreciated. Depreciation is recognized within each year as an expense, but it does not represent a cash expense. This is a concept that now enters into the statement of cash flows.

Exhibit 12–4 presents the current period cash flow. In effect, this statement takes the accrual basis statements and converts them to a cash flow for the period through a series of reconciling adjustments that account for the noncash amounts.

Understanding the cash/noncash concept makes sense of this statement. The starting point is the income from operations, the final item on the statement of revenue and expense. Depreciation and interest are added back, and changes in asset and liability accounts, both positive and negative, are recognized. These adjustments account for operating activities. Next, capital and related financing activities are addressed; then investing activities are adjusted. The result is a net increase in cash and cash equivalents of $45,000 in our example. This figure is added to the cash balance at the beginning of the

year ($145,000) to arrive at the cash balance at the end of the year ($190,000). Now refer back to the balance sheet, and you will find the cash balance is indeed $190,000. So the fourth major report—the statement of cash flows—interlocks with the other three major reports.

SUBSIDIARY REPORTS

The subsidiary reports are just that: subsidiary to the major reports. These reports support the major reports by providing more detail. For example, patient service revenue totals on the statement of revenue and expenses are often expanded in more detail on a subsidiary report. The same thing is true of operating expense. These reports are called "schedules" instead of "statements"—a sure sign that they are subsidiary reports.

SUMMARY

The four major reports fit together; each makes its own contribution to the whole. A checklist for balance sheet review (Exhibit 12–5) and a checklist for review of the statement of revenue and expense (Exhibit 12–6) are provided.

Exhibit 12–4 Westside Clinic Statement of Cash Flows

Statement of Cash Flows	For the Year Ending	
	December 31, 20x2	December 31, 20x1
Operating Activities		
Income from operations	$115,000	$50,000
Adjustments to reconcile income from operations to net cash flows from operating activities		
Depreciation and amortization	40,000	40,000
Interest expense	20,000	24,000
Changes in asset and liability accounts		
Patient accounts receivable	50,000	(250,000)
Inventories	(5,000)	(5,000)
Prepaid expenses and other assets	(2,000)	(1,000)
Accounts payable and accrued expenses	(9,000)	185,000
Net cash flow from operating activities	$209,000	$43,000
Cash Flows from Noncapital Financing Activities	0	0
Cash Flows from Capital and Related Financing Activities		
Acquisition of equipment	$0	$(300,000)
Proceeds from loan for equipment	0	300,000
Interest paid on long-term obligations	(20,000)	0
Repayment of long-term obligations	(48,000)	0
Net cash flows from capital and related financing activities	(68,000)	0
Cash Flows from Investing Activities		
Interest income received	$5,000	$2,000
Investments purchased (net)	(101,000)	0
Net cash flows from investing activities	(96,000)	2,000
Net Increase (Decrease) in Cash and Cash Equivalents	$45,000	$45,000
Cash and Cash Equivalents, Beginning of Year	145,000	100,000
Cash and Cash Equivalents, End of Year	$190,000	$145,000

Courtesy of Resource Group, Ltd., Dallas, Texas.

Exhibit 12–5 Checklist for Balance Sheet Review

1. What is the date on the balance sheet?
2. Are there large discrepancies in balances between the prior year and the current year?
3. Did total assets increase over the prior year?
4. Did current assets increase, decrease, or stay about the same?
5. Did current liabilities increase, decrease, or stay about the same?
6. Did land, plant, and equipment increase or decrease significantly over the prior year?
7. Did long-term debt increase or decrease significantly over the prior year?

Exhibit 12–6 Checklist for Review of the Statement of Revenue and Expense

1. What is the period reported on the statement of revenue and expense?
2. Is it one year or a shorter period? If it is a shorter period, why is that?
3. Are there large discrepancies in balances between the prior year operations and the current year operations?
4. Did total operating revenue increase over the prior year?
5. Did total operating expenses increase, decrease, or stay about the same? Is any particular line item unusually large or small?
6. Did income from operations increase, decrease, or stay about the same?
7. Are there unusual nonoperating gains or losses?
8. Did the current year result in an excess of revenue over expense? Is it as much as the prior year?
9. Did long-term debt increase or decrease significantly over the prior year?

 INFORMATION CHECKPOINT

What Is Needed?	A set of financial statements, ideally containing the four major reports plus subsidiary reports for additional detail.
Where Is It Found?	Possibly in the files of your supervisor, or in the finance offices, or the office of the administrator.
How Is It Used?	Study the financial statement to see how they fit together; use the checklists included in this chapter to assist in your review. Understanding how the statements work will give you another valuable managerial tool.

KEY TERMS

Accrual Basis of Accounting
Balance Sheet
Cash Basis of Accounting
Statement of Revenue and Expense
Statement of Cash Flows
Statement of Fund Balance/Net Worth
Subsidiary Reports

 DISCUSSION QUESTIONS

1. Can you give an example of an asset? A liability?
2. Does the concept of revenue less expense equaling an increase in equity or fund balance make sense to you? If not, why not?
3. Are you familiar with the current maturity of long-term debt? What example of it can you give in your own life (either at work or at home)?
4. Do you get a chance to review financial statements at your place of work? Would you like to? Why?

CHAPTER 13

Financial and Operating Ratios as Performance Measures

THE IMPORTANCE OF RATIOS

Ratios are convenient and uniform measures that are widely adopted in health care financial management. They are important because they are so widely used. And they are especially important because they are used for credit analysis. But a ratio is only a number. It has to be considered within the context of the operation. There is another caveat: ratio analysis should be conducted as a comparative analysis. In other words, one ratio standing alone with nothing to compare it to does not mean very much. When interpreting ratios, the differences between periods must be considered, and the reasons for such differences should be sought. It is a good

practice to compare results to equivalent computations from outside the organization—regional figures from similar institutions would be a good example of such outside sources. Caution and good managerial judgment must always be exercised when working with ratios.

Financial ratios basically pull together two elements of the financial statements: one expressed as the numerator and one as the denominator. To calculate a ratio, divide the bottom number (the denominator) into the top number (the numerator). Mini-Case Study 1 in Chapter 16 uses financial ratios as indicators of financial position and for purposes of credit analysis. We highly recommend that you spend time with Mini-Case Study 1, as it will add depth and background to the contents of this chapter.

In this chapter we will examine liquidity, solvency, and profitability ratios. Exhibit 13–1 sets out eight basic ratios that are widely used in health care organizations: four liquidity types, two solvency types, and two profitability types. All are discussed below.

LIQUIDITY RATIOS

Liquidity ratios reflect the ability of the organization to meet its current obligations. Li-

Exhibit 13–1 Eight Basic Ratios Used in Health Care

Liquidity Ratios
1. Current Ratio

$$\frac{\text{Current Assets}}{\text{Current Liabilities}}$$

2. Quick Ratio

$$\frac{\text{Cash and Cash Equivalents } + \text{ Net Receivables}}{\text{Current Liabilities}}$$

3. Days Cash on Hand (DCOH)

$$\frac{\text{Unrestricted Cash and Cash Equivalents}}{\text{Cash Operation Expenses} \div \text{No. of Days in Period (365)}}$$

4. Days Receivables

$$\frac{\text{Net Receivables}}{\text{Net Credit Revenues} \div \text{No. of Days in Period (365)}}$$

Solvency Ratios
5. Debt Service Coverage Ratio (DSCR)

$$\frac{\text{Change in Unrestricted Net Assets (net income)} + \text{Interest, Depreciation, Amortization}}{\text{Maximum Annual Debt Service}}$$

6. Liabilities to Fund Balance

$$\frac{\text{Total Liabilities}}{\text{Unrestricted Fund Balances}}$$

Profitability Ratios
7. Operating Margin (%)

$$\frac{\text{Operating Income (Loss)}}{\text{Total Operating Revenues}}$$

8. Return on Total Assets (%)

$$\frac{\text{EBIT (Earnings before Interest and Taxes)}}{\text{Total Assets}}$$

Courtesy of Resource Group, Ltd., Dallas, Texas.

quidity ratios measure short-term sufficiency. As the name implies, they measure the ability of the organization to "be liquid": in other words, to have sufficient cash—or assets that can be converted to cash—on hand.

Current Ratio

The current ratio equals current assets divided by current liabilities. To use the Westside Clinic example in the previous chapter,

$$\frac{\text{Current Assets}}{\text{Current Liabilities}} = \frac{\$120,000}{\$60,000} = 2 \text{ to } 1$$

This ratio is considered to be a measure of short-term debt-paying ability. However, it must be carefully interpreted. The standard by which current ratio is measured is 2 to 1, as computed above.

Quick Ratio

The quick ratio equals cash plus short-term investments plus net receivables divided by current liabilities. In our example,

$$\frac{\text{Cash and Cash Equivalents} + \text{Net Receivables}}{\text{Current Liabilities}} \quad \frac{\$65,000}{\$60,000} = 1.08 \text{ to } 1$$

The standard by which the quick ratio is measured is generally 1 to 1. The computation above, at 1.08 to 1, is a little better than the standard.

This ratio is considered to be an even more severe test of short-term debt-paying ability (even more than the current ratio). The quick ratio is also known as the acid-test ratio, for obvious reasons.

Days Cash on Hand

The days cash on hand (DCOH) equals unrestricted cash and investments divided by cash operating expenses/365. In our example,

$$\frac{\text{Unrestricted Cash and Cash Equivalents}}{\text{Cash Operating Expenses} \div \text{No. of Days in Period}} \quad \frac{\$330,000}{\$11,000} = 30 \text{ days}$$

There is no concrete standard for this computation.

This ratio indicates cash on hand in relation to the amount of daily operating expense. The example above indicates the organization has 30 days worth of operating expenses represented in the amount of (unrestricted) cash on hand.

Days Receivables

The days receivables computation is represented as net receivables divided by net credit revenues/365. In our example,

$$\frac{\text{Net Receivables}}{\text{Net Credit Revenue}/\text{No. of Days in Period}} = \frac{\$720,000}{\$12,000} = 60 \text{ days}$$

This computation represents the number of days in receivables. The older a receivable is, the more difficult it becomes to collect. Therefore, this computation is a measure of worth as well as performance.

There is no hard and fast rule for this computation because much depends on the mix of payers in your organization. The example above indicates that the organization has 60 days' worth of credit revenue tied up in net receivables. This computation is a common measure of billing and collection performance. There are many "days receivables" regional and national figures to compare to your own organization's computation.

Figure 13–1 shows how the information for the numerator and the denominator of each calculation is obtained. It takes the Westside Clinic balance sheet and the statement of revenue and expense that were discussed in the preceding chapter and illustrates the source of each figure in the four ratios just discussed. The multiple computations for days cash on hand and for days receivables are further broken down into a three-step process. If you study Figure 13–1 and work with Mini-Case Study 1, you will own this process.

SOLVENCY RATIOS

Solvency ratios reflect the ability of the organization to pay the annual interest and principal obligations on its long-term debt. As the name implies, they measure the ability of the organization to "be solvent": in other words,

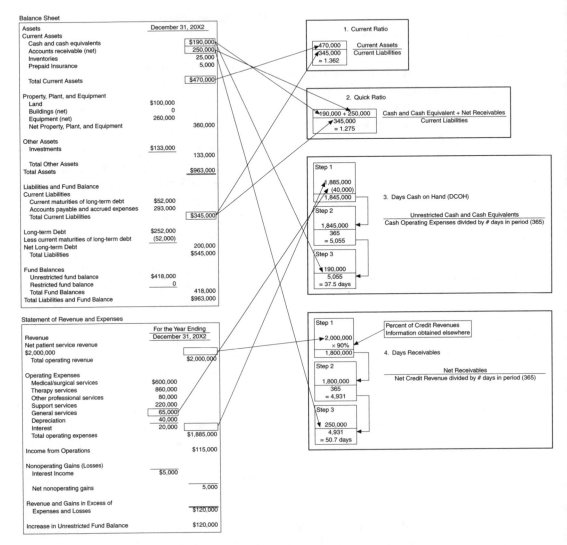

Figure 13–1 Examples of Liquidity Ratio Calculations. Courtesy of Resource Group, Ltd., Dallas, Texas.

to have sufficient resources to meet its long-term obligations.

Debt Service Coverage Ratio

The debt service coverage ratio (DSCR) is represented as change in unrestricted net assets (net income) plus interest, depreciation, and amortization divided by maximum annual debt service. In our example,

$$\frac{\text{Change in Unrestricted Net Assets (Net Income)} + \text{Interest, Depreciation, and Amortization}}{\text{Maximum Annual Debt Service}} = \frac{\$250,000}{\$100,000} = 2.5$$

This ratio is universally used in credit analysis and figures prominently in Mini-Case Study 1.

Each lending institution has its particular criteria for the DSCR. Lending agreements often have a provision that requires the DSCR to be maintained at or above a certain figure.

Liabilities To Fund Balance (or Debt to Net Worth)

The liabilities to fund balance or net worth computation is represented as total liabilities divided by unrestricted net assets (i.e., fund balances or net worth), or total debt divided by tangible net worth. In our example,

$$\frac{\text{Total Liabilities}}{\text{Unrestricted Fund Balances}} = \frac{\$2,000,000}{\$2,250,000} = .80$$

This figure is a quick indicator of debt load.

Another indicator that is more severe is long-term debt to net worth (fund balance), which is computed as long-term debt divided by fund balance. This computation is somewhat equivalent to the quick ratio discussed above in its restrictiveness to net worth computation.

A mirror image of total liabilities to fund balance is total assets to fund balance, which is computed as total assets divided by fund balance.

Figure 13–2 shows how the information for the numerator and the denominator of each calculation is obtained. This figure again takes the Westside Clinic balance sheet and statement of revenue and expense that were discussed in the preceding chapter and illustrates the source of each figure in the two solvency ratios just discussed, along with each figure in the two profitability ratios still to be discussed. When multiple computations are necessary, they are further broken down into a two-step process.

PROFITABILITY RATIOS

Profitability ratios reflect the ability of the organization to operate with an excess of operating revenue over operating expense. Non-profit organizations may not call this result a profit, but the measurement ratios are still generally called profitability ratios, whether they are applied to for-profit or nonprofit organizations.

Operating Margin

The operating margin, which is generally expressed as a percentage, is represented as operating income (loss) divided by total operating revenues. In our example,

$$\frac{\text{Operating Income (Loss)}}{\text{Total Operating Revenues}} = \frac{\$250,000}{\$5,000,000} = 5.0\%$$

This ratio is used for a number of managerial purposes and also sometimes enters into credit analysis. It is therefore a multipurpose measure. It is so universal that many outside sources are available for comparative purposes. The result of the computation must still be carefully considered because of variables in each period being compared.

Return on Total Assets

The return on total assets is represented as earnings before interest and taxes (EBIT) divided by total assets. In our example,

$$\frac{\text{EBIT}}{\text{Total Assets}} = \frac{\$400,000}{\$4,000,000} = 10\%$$

This is a broad measure in common use. Note the acronym *EBIT,* as its use is widespread in credit analysis circles.

This concludes the description of solvency and profitability ratios. Again, if you study Figure 13–2 and work with Mini-Case Study 1, you will own this process too.

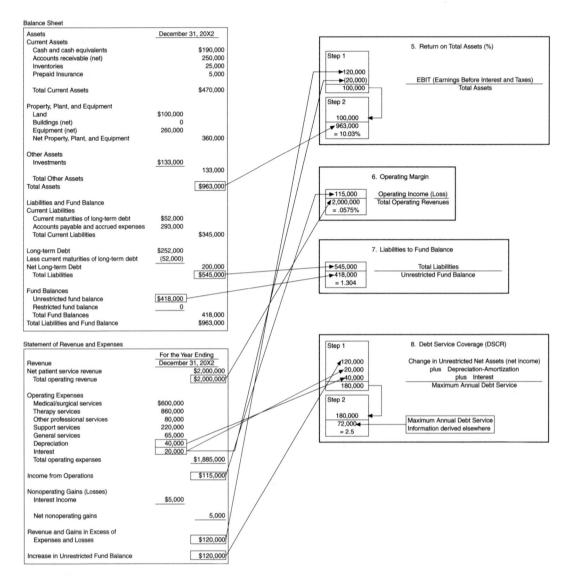

Figure 13–2 Examples of Solvency and Profitability Ratio Calculations. Courtesy of Resource Group, Ltd., Dallas, Texas.

INFORMATION CHECKPOINT

What Is Needed?	Reports that use ratios as measures.
Where Is It Found?	Possibly in your supervisor's file; in the administrator's office; in the chief executive officer's office.
How Is It Used?	Use as a measure against outside benchmarks (as discussed in this chapter); also use as internal benchmarks for departments/divisions/units; also use as benchmarks at various points over time.

KEY TERMS

Current Ratio
Days Cash on Hand (DCOH)
Days Receivables
Debt Service Coverage Ratio (DSCR)
Liabilities to Fund Balance
Liquidity Ratios
Operating Margin
Profitability Ratios
Quick Ratio
Return on Total Assets
Solvency Ratios

DISCUSSION QUESTIONS

1. Are there ratios in the reports you receive at your workplace?
2. If so, do you use them? How?
3. If not, do you believe ratios should be on the reports? Which reports?
4. Can you think of good outside sources that could be used to obtain ratios for comparative purposes? If the outside information was available, what ratios would you choose to use? Why?

CHAPTER 14

Other Types of Performance Measures

PROGRESS NOTES

After completing this chapter, you should be able to

1. Recognize performance measures that span a period of time.
2. Understand the concept of financial benchmarking.
3. Understand the use of the Pareto rule.
4. Compute quartiles for measurement purposes.

IMPORTANCE OF A VARIETY OF PERFORMANCE MEASURES

If operations are to be managed most effectively, a variety of performance measures must be in place for the organization. Generally a broad variety of such measures are available, and different organizations tend to lean toward using one type over another. One health care organization, for example, may rely heavily on one type of measure, whereas another organization may rely on a very different measurement profile. Generally speaking, a wider variety of performance measures

are evident in organizations that have adopted total quality improvement (TQI).

ADJUSTED PERFORMANCE MEASURES OVER TIME

We have previously discussed how measures over time are very effective. The example given in Figure 14–1 combines measures over time with a two-part case mix adjustment. (*Case mix adjustment* refers to adjusting for the acuity level of the patient. It may also refer to the level of resources required to provide care for the patient with the acuity level.) In this case, the desired measure is cost per discharge. The vertical axis is cost in dollars. The horizontal axis is time, a five-year span in this case. Two lines are plotted: the first is unadjusted for case mix, and the second is case mix adjusted. The unadjusted line rises over the five-year period. However, when the case mix adjustment is taken into account, the plotted line flattens out over time.

BENCHMARKING

Benchmarking is the continuous process of measuring products, services, and activities against the best levels of performance. These

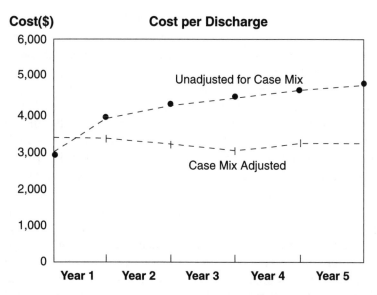

Figure 14–1 Adjusted Performance Measure over Time. *Source:* Reprinted from S.A. Finkler, *Cost Accounting for Health Care Organizations,* 2nd ed., p. 115, © 1999, Aspen Publishers, Inc.

best levels may be found inside the organization or outside it. Benchmarks are used to measure performance gaps.

There are three types of benchmarks:

1. A financial variable reported in an accounting system
2. A financial variable not reported in an accounting system
3. A nonfinancial variable.

How To Benchmark

The benchmarking methodology is predicated on the assumption that an exemplary process, similar to the process being examined, can be identified and examined to establish criteria for excellence. Benchmarking can be accomplished in one of several ways, including (1) studying the methods and end results of your prime competitors; (2) exam-

ining the analogous process of noncompetitors with a world-class reputation; or (3) analyzing processes within your own organization (or health system) that are worthy of being emulated. In any of these three cases, the necessary analysis will rely on one or both of the following methods: parametric analysis or process analysis. In parametric analysis the characteristics or attributes of similar services or products are examined. In process analysis the process that serves as a standard for comparison is examined in detail to learn how and why it performs the way it does.

Benchmarking is used for opportunity assessment. Opportunity assessment, utilized for strategic planning and for process engineering, provides information about the way things should or possibly could be. Benchmarking is a primary information-gathering approach for opportunity assessment when it is used in this way.

Benchmarking in Health Care

Financial benchmarking compares financial measures among benchmarking groups. This is the most common type of "peer group" health care benchmarking in use. An example of a health care financial benchmarking report is provided in Table 14–1. The computation of ratios included in this report has been discussed in the preceding chapter. The computation of quartiles is described later in this chapter.

Statistical benchmarking is a related method of benchmarking. In this case, the statistics of utilization and service delivery, upon which inflow and outflow are based, are compared to those of certain other hospitals. An example of statistical information available for this type of benchmarking is given in Exhibit 14–1. This exhibit sets out number of acute care beds and total available bed days (number of beds times 365 days in a full year equals total available bed days). Total bed days are then compared to actual patient days (called "reported patient days" in this report). The result of the comparison is the occupancy percentage for the applicable period. (Computation of the occupancy percentage is accomplished by dividing patient days by bed days; in the case of the first line item, 8,192 divided by 17,836 equals a 45.93 percent occupancy rate.) The information is provided for a quarter (April through June) and for a full year (12-month totals). Line-item information is provided for all hospitals in district 8. (Florida regulatory health care reporting is divided into 11 districts for control purposes. Each district is then divided into a series of subdistricts.) At the bottom of the report, totals by subdistrict are included, along with a district total.

In summary, benchmarking is a comparative method that allows an overview of the individual organization's indicators. Objective measurement criteria are always required for best practices purposes.

Table 14–1 Financial Benchmark Example

Indicator	Total	Upper Quartile	Mid-Quartile	Low Quartile
No. of hospitals	500.0	105.0	305.0	90.0
Total margin (%)	4.1	11.0	4.5	–6.0
Occupancy (%)	64.5	65.7	64.0	56.1
Deductions from GPR (%)	29.0	28.5	29.2	31.3
Medicare (%GPR)	53.0	55.1	52.2	50.4
Medicaid (%GPR)	10.0	8.4	9.7	13.7
Self-pay (%GPR)	7.0	8.5	7.1	6.4
Managed care plans (%GPR)*	16.0	13.0	17.0	17.5
Other third party (%GPR)	14.0	15.0	14.0	12.0
Outpatient revenue (%GPR)	22.0	25.0	21.8	17.7
No. of days in accounts receivable	75.0	70.0	74.0	80.0
Cash flow as a percentage of total debt	30.0	60.0	27.0	–0.5
Long-Term Debt as a Percentage of total assets	35.0	26.0	36.0	42.0
Change in admissions (1993–1997, %)	–7.0	–3.7	–6.3	–15.8
Change in inpatient days (1993–1997, %)	–6.0	–1.8	–6.5	–11.1

*Note: Managed care plans other than Title XVIII or Title XIX. All amounts are fictitious.

Source: Reprinted from J.J. Baker, *Activity-Based Costing and Activity-Based Management for Health Care*, p. 140, © 1998, Aspen Publishers, Inc.

Exhibit 14–1 Hospital Bed and Service Utilization by District

Agency for Health Care Administration
January 1999 Hospital Bed Need Projections
Acute Care Utilization by District, Subdistrict, and Facility for July 1997–June 1998 (excluding LTC Hospital Beds and Neonatal Level II and III Beds)

Sub-dist.	County	Fac. ID	Name of Facility	APR–JUN 1998				12 MONTH TOTALS		
				Acute Care Beds	Total Beddays	Rptd. Patient Days	Occup./ Quarter (%)	Total Beddays	Total Patient Days	Occup. (%)
DISTRICT 8										
1	Charlotte	100236	FAWCETT MEMORIAL HOSPITAL	196	17,836	8,192	45.93%	73,242	35,998	49.15%
1	Charlotte	100047	CHARLOTTE REGIONAL MEDICAL CENTER	156	14,196	6,446	45.41%	56,940	25,985	45.64%
1	Charlotte	100077	ST JOSEPH HOSP OF PORT CHARLOTTE	202	18,472	7,866	42.58%	76,560	34,697	45.32%
2	Collier	100018	NAPLES COMMUNITY HOSPITAL	331	30,121	19,413	64.45%	120,815	80,519	66.65%
2	Collier	120006	NORTH COLLIER HOSPITAL	50	4,550	4,179	91.85%	18,250	17,121	93.81%
3	Desoto	100175	DESOTO MEMORIAL HOSPITAL	82	7,462	2,117	28.37%	29,930	9,313	31.12%
4	Hendry	100098	HENDRY REGIONAL MEDICAL CENTER	66	6,006	860	14.32%	24,090	4,380	18.18%
5	Lee	100244	CAPE CORAL HOSPITAL	281	25,571	9,867	38.59%	102,565	41,630	40.59%
5	Lee	100107	EAST POINTE HOSPITAL	75	6,825	2,029	29.73%	27,375	9,026	32.97%
5	Lee	111522	GULF COAST HOSPITAL	110	10,010	3,025	30.22%	40,150	14,759	36.76%
5	Lee	100012	LEE MEMORIAL HOSP.-CLEVELAND	367	33,397	13,346	39.96%	133,955	55,305	41.29%
5	Lee	120005	LEE MEMORIAL HOSP.-HEALTHPARK	180	16,380	11,305	69.02%	65,700	45,510	69.27%
5	Lee	100220	SOUTHWEST FLORIDA REG. MEDICAL CTR.	380	34,580	11,372	32.89%	138,700	57,984	41.81%
6	Sarasota	110004	ENGLEWOOD COMMUNITY HOSPITAL	90	8,190	4,396	53.68%	32,850	19,763	60.16%
6	Sarasota	100166	COLUMBIA DOCTORS HOSP. OF SARASOTA	147	13,377	9,414	70.37%	53,655	38,320	71.42%
6	Sarasota	100087	SARASOTA MEMORIAL (Bed conv. 1/22/98)	683	62,153	25,800	41.51%	249,926	110,033	44.03%
6	Sarasota	100070	BON SECOURS-VENICE HOSPITAL	276	25,116	12,443	49.54%	100,740	43,608	43.29%
			TOTALS Subdistrict 1 Total	554	50,504	22,504	44.56%	206,742	96,680	46.76%
			Subdistrict 2 Total	381	34,671	23,592	68.05%	139,065	97,640	70.21%
			Subdistrict 3 Total	82	7,462	2,117	28.37%	29,930	9,313	31.12%
			Subdistrict 4 Total	66	6,006	860	14.32%	24,090	4,380	18.18%
			Subdistrict 5 Total	1,393	126,763	50,944	40.19%	508,445	224,214	44.10%
			Subdistrict 6 Total	1,196	108,836	52,053	47.83%	437,171	211,724	48.43%
			DISTRICT 8 TOTAL	3,672	334,242	152,070	45.50%	1,345,443	643,951	47.86%

Source: Reprinted from *Florida Hospital Bed and Service Utilization by District, Utilization Data for July 1, 1997 Through June 30, 1998 to Support Florida Hospital Bed Need Projections for the January 1999 Batching Cycle*, p. 32, 1999, Agency for Health Care Administration, Tallahassee, Florida.

ECONOMIC MEASURES

Other performance measures may be made outside the actual confines of the facility. A good example of a widespread performance measure would be the role of community hospitals in the performance of local economies. Nonprofit organizations in particular are concerned about their ability to measure such performance. This case study gives a specific direction for such measurement efforts.

MEASUREMENT TOOLS

Pareto Analysis

Creating benchmarks, especially in an organization committed to continuous quality improvement, ultimately leads managers to exploring how to improve some step in a process. Pareto analysis is an analytical tool that employs the Pareto principle and helps in this exploration. Pareto was a 19th-century economist who was a pioneer in applying mathematics to economic theory. His Pareto principle states that 80 percent of an organization's problems, for example, are caused by 20 percent of the possible causes: thus the "80/20 Rule."

The usual way to display a Pareto analysis is through the construction of a Pareto diagram. A Pareto diagram displays the important causes of variation, as reflected in data collected on the causes of such variation. Figure 14–2 presents an example of a Pareto diagram. This example reinforces the idea behind the Pareto analysis: that the majority of problems are due to a small number of identifiable causes.

The chief financial officer of XYZZ Hospital believes that the billing and collection

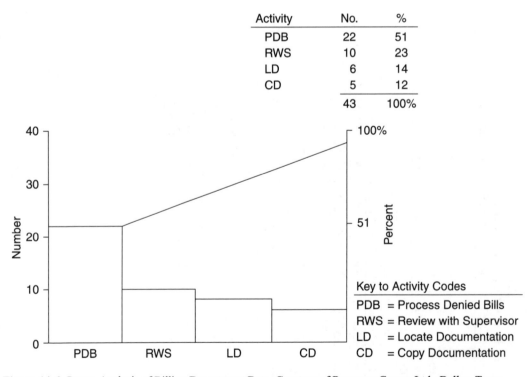

Figure 14–2 Pareto Analysis of Billing Department Data. Courtesy of Resource Group, Ltd., Dallas, Texas.

department is inefficient—or, to be more specific, that the process is probably inefficient. An activity analysis is conducted. It shows that billing personnel are spending much time on unproductive work. This Pareto diagram displays the activities involved in resubmitting denied bills. (Resubmitting denied bills is an inefficient and nonproductive activity, as we have discussed in a preceding chapter.)

Constructing a Pareto diagram is really simple. The first step is to prepare a table that shows the activities recorded, the numbers of times the activities were observed, and the percentage of the total number of times represented by each count. In Figure 14–2, the total number of times these activities were observed is 43. The number of times that processing denied bills for resubmission (coded as PDB) was observed is 22. Thus, 100 (22/43) = 51 percent. Similar calculations complete the table. The table of observations is shown in its entirety within the exhibit.

The Pareto diagram has two vertical axes, the left one corresponding to the "No." column in the table, the right one corresponding to the "%" column in the table. On the horizontal axis, the activities are listed, creating bases of equal length for the rectangles shown in the diagram. The activities are listed in decreasing order of occurrence. Constructing the diagram in this manner means that the most frequently observed activity lies on the left extreme of the diagram and the least frequently observed activity on the right extreme. The heights of the rectangles are drawn to show the frequencies of the activities, and then the sides of the rectangle are drawn.

The next step is to locate the cumulative percentage of the activities, using the right-hand axis. The cumulative percent for the first rectangle, labeled *PDB*, is 51 percent. (The calculation of the 51 percent was previ-

ously explained.) For the second rectangle from the left, labeled *RWS,* the cumulative percentage is 51 + 23 = 74 percent. The 74 percent is plotted over the right-hand side of the rectangle labeled *RWS.* The next cumulative percentage, for the third rectangle from the left, labeled *LD,* is 51 + 23 + 14 = 88 percent. The 88 percent is plotted over the right-hand side of the rectangle labeled *LD.* The last cumulative percentage is, of course, 100 percent (51 + 23 + 14 + 12 = 100 percent), and it is plotted over the right-hand side of the last rectangle on the right, labeled *CD.*

Now draw straight lines between the plotted cumulative percentages as shown in the exhibit. The next step is to label the axes and add a title to the diagram. In Figure 14–2, the tallest rectangle could be lightly shaded to highlight the most frequent activity, suggesting the one that may deserve first priority in problem solving.

In general, the activities requiring priority attention, the "vital few," will appear on the left of the diagram where the slope of the curve is steepest. Pareto diagrams are often constructed before and after improvement efforts for comparative purposes. When comparing before and after, if the improvement measures are effective either the order of the bars will change or the curve will be much flatter.

In conclusion, note that many authorities recommend that Pareto analysis take the *costs* of the activities into account. The concern is that a very frequent problem may nevertheless imply less overall cost than a relatively rare but disastrous problem. Also, before basing a Pareto analysis on frequencies, as this example does, the analyst needs to decide that the seriousness of the problem is roughly proportional to the frequency. If seriousness fails to satisfy this criterion, then activities should be measured in some other way. Figure 14–2 underlines the importance of judging the relevance of the measurements used in a Pareto analysis.

Quartile Computation

Reporting by quartiles is an effective way to show ranges of either financial or statistical results. Quartiles represent a distribution into four classes, each of which contains one quarter of the whole. Each of the four classes is a quartile. Quartile computation is not very complicated, although several steps are involved. We can use the outpatient revenue line item in Table 14–1 to illustrate the computation of quartile data. (Outpatient revenue, expressed as a percentage of all revenue, is found on the tenth line down from the top in Table 14–1.) We see from the first line that 500 hospitals were in the group used for benchmarking. The median is found for the outpatient revenue of the entire group of hospitals. (Most computer spreadsheet programs offer median computation as an available function.) Then each hospital's revenue is identified as a percentage of this median.

These percentages are arrayed. In the case of this report, cutoffs were then made to arrange the arrayed percentages into three groups. The percentages that were between 0 and 25 percent were designated as the low-quartile group. The percentages that were between 75 and 100 percent were designated as the high-quartile group. The percentages that were between 25 and 75 percent were designated as the midquartile group.

The average (also known as the arithmetic mean) of each quartile group is then presented in this report. Thus, the outpatient revenue (expressed as a percentage of gross revenue) for the upper-quartile group in the report is 25.0; for the middle-quartile group, 21.8; and for the low-quartile group, 17.7. (Note that a grand total of the entire 500 hospitals is also computed and presented in the left-hand column; the grand total amounts to 22 percent.) In summary, quartiles are based on a quantitative method of computation and are an effective way to illustrate a variety of performance measures.

 INFORMATION CHECKPOINT

What Is Needed?   Examples of performance measures used in your organization.
Where Is It Found?   This information is probably found in the quality assurance department.
How Is It Used?   Used to measure employee performance or departmental/division/unit performance. Many different measures; application in many ways. Can be either clinical or financial measures.

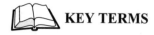 **KEY TERMS**

Benchmarking
Case Mix Adjusted
Pareto Analysis
Performance
Performance Measures
Quartiles

DISCUSSION QUESTIONS

1. Does your organization use measurements such as case mix adjustment over time?
2. If not, do you believe it should? Why?
3. Does your organization use financial benchmarking?
4. Would you use it if you had a chance to do so? Why?

PART IV

Case Study

CHAPTER 15

Case Study: Metropolis Health System

BACKGROUND

1. The Hospital System

Metropolis Health System (MHS) offers comprehensive health care services. It is a midsize taxing district hospital. Although MHS has the power to raise revenues through taxes, it has not done so for the past seven years.

2. The Area

MHS is located in the town of Metropolis, which has a population of 50,000. The town has a small college and a modest number of environmentally clean industries.

3. Metropolis Health System Services

MHS has taken significant steps to reduce hospital stays. It has developed a comprehensive array of services that are accessible, cost-effective, and responsive to the community's needs. These services are wellness oriented in that they strive for prevention rather than treatment. As a result of these steps, inpatient visits have increased overall by only 1,000 per year since 1998, whereas outpatient/same-day surgery visits have had an increase of over 50,000 per year.

A number of programmatic, service, and facility enhancements support this major transition in the community's institutional health care. They are geared to provide the quality, convenience, affordability, and personal care that best suit the health needs of the people whom MHS serves.

- *Rehabilitation and Wellness Center*—for outpatient physical therapy and return-to-work services plus cardiac and pulmonary rehabilitation to get people back to a normal way of living.
- *Home Health Services*—bringing skilled care, therapy, and medical social services into the home; a comfortable and affordable alternative in longer term care.
- *Same-Day Surgery (SDS)*—eliminating the need for an overnight stay. Since 1998, same-day surgery procedures have doubled at MHS.
- *Skilled Nursing Facility*—inpatient service to assist patients in returning more fully to an independent lifestyle.
- *Community Health and Wellness*—community health outreach programs that provide educational seminars on a variety of health issues, a diabetes education center, support services for patients with cancer, health awareness events, and a women's health resource center.

- *Occupational Health Services (OH)*—helping to reduce workplace injury costs at over 100 area businesses through consultation on injury avoidance and work-specific rehabilitation services.
- *Recovery Services*—offering mental health services including substance abuse programs and support groups along with individual and family counseling.

4. Metropolis Health Systems Plant

The central building for the hospital is in the center of a two–square block area. A physicians' office building is to the west. Two administrative offices, converted from former residences, are on one corner. The new ambulatory center, completed two years ago, has an "L" shape and sits on one corner of the western block. A laundry and maintenance building sits on the extreme back of the property. A four-story parking garage is located on the eastern back corner. An employee parking lot sits beside the laundry and maintenance building. Visitor parking lots fill the front eastern portion of the property. A helipad is on the extreme western edge of the property behind the physicians' office building.

5. MHS Board of Trustees

MHS is governed by 8 local community leaders who bring diverse skills to the board. The trustees generously volunteer their time to plan the strategic direction of MHS, thus ensuring the system's ability to provide quality comprehensive health care to the community.

6. MHS Management

MHS is managed by a chief executive officer. Seven senior vice presidents report to the CEO. MHS is organized into 23 major responsibility centers.

7. MHS Employees

All 500 team members employed by MHS are integral to achieving the high standards for which the system strives. The quality improvement (QI) program, implemented in 1995, is aimed at meeting client needs sooner, better, and more cost-effectively. Participants in the program are from all areas of the system.

8. MHS Physicians

The MHS medical staff are a key part of MHS's ability to provide excellence in health care. Over 75 physicians cover more than 30 medical specialties. The high quality of their training and their commitment to the practice of medicine are great assets to the health of the community.

The physicians are very much a part of MHS's drive for continual improvement upon the quality health care services offered in the community. MHS brings in medical experts from around the country to provide training in new techniques, made possible by MHS's technological advancements. MHS also ensures that physicians are offered seminars, symposiums, and continuing education programs that permit them to remain current with changes in the medical field.

The medical staff's quality improvement program has begun a care path initiative to track effective means for diagnosis, treatment, and follow-up. This initiative will help avoid unnecessary or duplicate use of expensive medications or technologies.

9. MHS Foundation

Metropolis Health Foundation is presently being created to serve as the philanthropic arm of MHS. It will operate in a separate corporation governed by a board of 12 community leaders and supported by a 15-member special events board. The mission of the foundation will be to secure financial and nonfinancial support for realizing the MHS vision of providing comprehensive health care for the community.

Funds donated by individuals, businesses, foundations, and organizations will be designated for a variety of purposes at MHS, including the operations of specific departments, community outreach programs, continuing education for employees, endowment, equipment, and capital improvements.

10. MHS Volunteer Auxiliary

There are 500 volunteers who provide over 60,000 hours of service to MHS each year. These men and women assist in virtually every part of the system's operations. They also conduct community programs on behalf of MHS.

The auxiliary funds its programs and makes financial contributions to MHS through money it raises on renting televisions and vending gifts and other items at the hospital. In the past, its donations to MHS have generally been designated for medical equipment purchases. The auxiliary has given $250,000 over the last five years.

11. Planning the Future for MHS

The Metropolis Health System has identified five areas of desired service and programmatic enhancement in its five-year strategic plan:

1. Ambulatory Services
2. Physical Medicine and Rehabilitative Services
3. Cardiovascular Services
4. Oncology Services
5. Community Health Services

MHS has set out to answer the most critical health needs that are specific to its community. Over the next five years, the MHS strategic plan will continue a tradition of quality, community-oriented health care to meet future demands.

12. Financing the Future

Metropolis Health System has established a corporate depreciation fund. The fund's purpose is to ease the financial burden of replacing fixed assets. Presently, it has almost $2 million for needed equipment or renovations.

I. METROPOLIS HEALTH SYSTEM CASE STUDY

Financial Statements

- Balance Sheet (Exhibit 15–1)
- Statement of Revenue and Expense (Exhibit 15–2)
- Statement of Cash Flows (Exhibit 15–3)
- Statement of Changes in Fund Balance (Exhibit 15–4)
- Schedule of Property, Plant, and Equipment (Exhibit 15–5)
- Schedule of Patient Revenue (Exhibit 15–6)
- Schedule of Operating Expenses (Exhibit 15–7)

Statistics and Organizational Structure

- Statistics (Exhibit 15–8)
- MHS Nursing Practice and Administration Organization Chart (Figure 15–1)
- MHS Executive-Level Organization Chart (Figure 15–2)

Variance Analysis Report and Recommendations

- Radiology Diagnostic Clinic Report

Exhibit 15–1 Balance Sheet

Metropolis Health System
Balance Sheet
March 31, 2000

Assets		Liabilities and Fund Balance	
		Current Liabilities	
Current Assets			
Cash and Cash Equivalents	$1,150,000	Current Maturities of Long-Term	
Assets Whose Use Is Limited	825,000	Debt	525,000
Patient Accounts Receivable	7,400,000	Accounts Payable and Accrued	
(Net of $1,300,000 Allowance		Expenses	$4,900,000
for Bad Debts)		Bond Interest Payable	300,000
		Reimbursement Settlement	
Other Receivables	150,000	Payable	100,000
Inventories	900,000	Total Current Liabilities	5,825,000
Prepaid Expenses	200,000		
		Long-Term Debt	6,000,000
Total Current Assets	10,625,000	Less Current Portion of	
		Long-Term Debt	<525,000>
Assets Whose Use Is Limited		Net Long-Term Debt	5,475,000
Corporate Funded Depreciation	1,950,000		
Held by Trustee Under Bond		Total Liabilities	11,300,000
Indenture Agreement	1,425,000		
		Fund Balances	
Total Assets Whose Use Is		General Fund	21,500,000
Limited	3,375,000		
		Total Fund Balances	21,500,000
Less Current Portion	<825,000>		
		Total Liabilities and Fund	
Net Assets Whose Use Is Limited	2,550,000	Balances	32,800,000
Property, Plant, and Equipment, net	19,300,000		
Other Assets	325,000		
Total Assets	$32,800,000		

Exhibit 15–2 Statement of Revenue and Expense

Metropolis Health System
Statement of Revenue and Expense
For the Year Ended March 31, 2000

Revenue
Net patient service revenue	$34,000,000	
Other revenue	1,100,000	
Total Operating Revenue		$35,100,000

Expenses
Nursing services	$5,025,000	
Other professional services	13,100,000	
General services	3,200,000	
Support services	8,300,000	
Depreciation	1,900,000	
Amortization	50,000	
Interest	325,000	
Provision for doubtful accounts	1,500,000	
Total Expenses		33,400,000
Income from Operations		$1,700,000

Nonoperating Gains (Losses)
Unrestricted gifts and memorials	$20,000	
Interest income	80,000	
Nonoperating Gains, Net		100,000
Revenue and Gains in Excess of Expenses and Losses		$1,800,000

Exhibit 15–3 Statement of Cash Flows

Metropolis Health System
Statement of Cash Flows
For the Year Ended March 31, 2000

Statement of Cash Flows

Operating Activities	
Income from operations	$1,700,000
Adjustments to reconcile income from operations to net cash flows from operating activities	
Depreciation and amortization	1,950,000
Changes in asset and liability accounts	
Patient accounts receivable	250,000
Other receivables	<50,000>
Inventories	<50,000>
Prepaid expenses and other assets	<50,000>
Accounts payable and accrued expenses	<400,000>
Reduction of bond interest payable	<25,000>
Estimated third-party payer settlements	<75,000>
Interest income received	80,000
Unrestricted gifts and memorials received	20,000
Net cash flow from operating activities	$3,350,000
Cash Flows from Capital and Related Financing Activities	
Repayment of long-term obligations	<500,000>
Cash Flows from Investing Activities	
Purchase of assets whose use is limited	<100,000>
Equipment purchases and building improvements	<2,000,000>
Net Increase (Decrease) in Cash and Cash Equivalents	$750,000
Cash and Cash Equivalents, Beginning of Year	400,000
Cash and Cash Equivalents, End of Year	$1,150,000

Exhibit 15–4 Statement of Changes in Fund Balance

Metropolis Health System Statement of Changes in Fund Balance For the Year Ended March 31, 2000	
General Fund Balance April 1, 1999	$19,700,000
Revenue and Gains in Excess of Expenses and Losses	1,800,000
General Fund Balance March 31, 2000	$21,500,000

Exhibit 15–5 Schedule of Property, Plant, and Equipment

Metropolis Health System Schedule of Property, Plant, and Equipment For the Year Ended March 31, 2000	
Buildings and Improvements	$14,700,000
Land Improvements	1,100,000
Equipment	28,900,000
Total	$44,700,000
Less Accumulated Depreciation	(26,100,000)
Net Depreciable Assets	$18,600,000
Land	480,000
Construction in Progress	220,000
Net Property, Plant, and Equipment	$19,300,000

Exhibit 15–6 Schedule of Patient Revenue

Metropolis Health System
Schedule of Patient Revenue
For the Year Ended March 31, 2000

Patient Services Revenue	
Routine revenue	$9,850,000
Laboratory	7,375,000
Radiology and CT scanner	5,825,000
OB–nursery	450,000
Pharmacy	3,175,000
Emergency service	2,200,000
Medical and surgical supply and IV	5,050,000
Operating rooms	5,250,000
Anesthesiology	1,600,000
Respiratory therapy	900,000
Physical therapy	1,475,000
EKG and EEG	1,050,000
Ambulance service	900,000
Oxygen	575,000
Home health and hospice	1,675,000
Substance abuse	375,000
Other	775,000
Subtotal	$48,500,000
Less allowances and charity care	14,500,000
Net Patient Service Revenue	$34,000,000

Exhibit 15–7 Schedule of Operating Expenses

Metropolis Health System
Schedule of Operating Expenses
For the Year Ended March 31, 2000

Nursing Services		General Services	
Routine Medical-Surgical	$3,880,000	Dietary	$1,055,000
Operating Room	300,000	Maintenance	1,000,000
Intensive Care Units	395,000	Laundry	295,000
OB-Nursery	150,000	Housekeeping	470,000
Other	300,000	Security	50,000
Total	$5,025,000	Medical Records	330,000
		Total	$3,200,000
Other Professional Services			
Laboratory	$2,375,000	Support Services	
Radiology and CT Scanner	1,700,000	General	$4,600,000
Pharmacy	1,375,000	Insurance	240,000
Emergency Service	950,000	Payroll Taxes	1,130,000
Medical and Surgical Supply	1,800,000	Employee Welfare	1,900,000
Operating Rooms and Anesthesia	1,525,000	Other	430,000
Respiratory Therapy	525,000	Total	$8,300,000
Physical Therapy	700,000		
EKG and EEG	185,000	Depreciation	1,900,000
Ambulance Service	80,000	Amortization	50,000
Substance Abuse	460,000		
Home Health and Hospice	1,295,000		
Other	130,000	Interest Expense	325,000
Total	$13,100,000		
		Provision for Doubtful Accounts	1,500,000
		Total Operating Expenses	$33,400,000

Exhibit 15–8 Hospital Statistical Data

Metropolis Health System
Schedule of Hospital Statistics
For the Year Ended March 31, 2000

Inpatient Indicators: Departmental Volume Indicators:

Patient Days			
Medical and surgical	13650	Respiratory therapy treatments	51,480
Obstetrics	1080	Physical therapy treatments	34,050
Skilled nursing unit	4500	Laboratory workload units	
		(in thousands)	2,750
		EKGs	8,900
Admissions		CT scans	2,780
Adult acute care	3610	MRI scans	910
Newborn	315	Emergency room visits	11,820
Skilled nursing unit	440	Ambulance trips	2,320
		Home Health visits	14,950
Discharges			
Adult acute care	3580	Approximate number of employees	
Newborn	315	(FTE)	510
Skilled nursing unit	445		
Average Length of Stay (in days)	4.1		

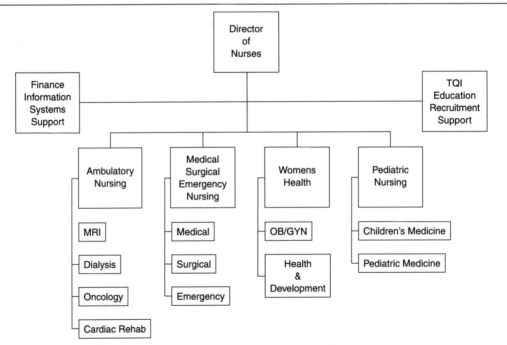

Figure 15–1 MHS Nursing Practice and Administration Organization Chart, Courtesy of Resource Group, Ltd., Dallas, Texas.

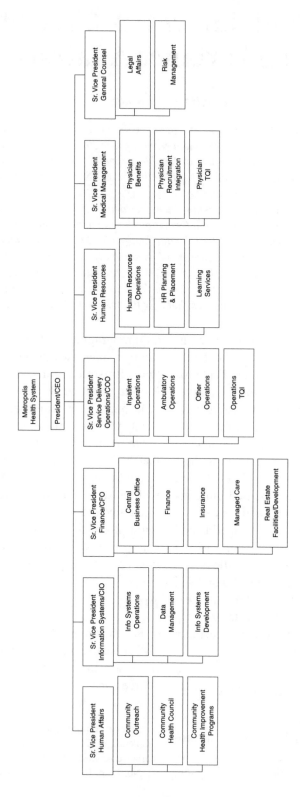

Figure 15–2 MHS Executive-Level Organization Chart. Courtesy of Resource Group, Ltd., Dallas, Texas.

Meeting the Challenge of Cost Containment: A Case Study Using Variance Analysis*

Cecilia L. Bautista

The Director of the MHS Radiology Diagnostic Clinic is Joseph Green. Joe has been at MHS for six months, having been recruited from a prestigious northeastern facility. His previous employer made extensive use of flexible budgeting and variance analysis. Joe believes he could do a better job managing the clinic at MHS if senior management would adopt a wider usage of flexible budgeting.

Joe arranges a meeting with his senior vice president, Mick Braun. To strengthen his case Joe brings along some supporting information. It is an article that his former boss had used when evaluating whether to adopt flexible budgeting. Mr. Braun's interest is sharpened when he sees the article contains a step-by-step analysis of the clinic's performance using a series of variance reports. He has been wanting better performance measures for the clinic. Maybe this approach is the answer. Joe and the vice president agree to meet again in two weeks. Mr. Braun promises that he will make a decision at that time.

Significant changes have taken place in the health care industry, including the development of government cost-containment programs, the additional competition for market share, and the evolution of alternative payment systems (i.e., managed care). Such changes have also brought about an immense shift in interest toward cost accounting. The changes have radically modified health care management practices and focused more attention on financial planning and control.

In this case study, the use of budgeting and variance analysis has been applied to the management of a radiology diagnostic clinic. A comparison of the clinic's 1992 budget and the actual costs incurred throughout the year will be presented, followed by a step-by-step analysis of the clinic's performance using a series of variance reports.

LRL RADIOLOGY DIAGNOSTIC CLINIC

The LRL Radiology Diagnostic Clinic provides a wide range of diagnostic services, including fluoroscopic, ultrasonographic, and mammographic studies. It contains four X-ray machines, two mammography units, and two ultrasound units. The clinic operates Monday through Friday from 9:00 a.m. to 7:00 p.m., with radiologists available from 10:00 a.m. to 6:00 p.m.

On average, the clinic performs approximately 60,000 imaging procedures per year. It caters to approximately 42,875 clients yearly, with close to 1.4 procedures done per client. The clinic caters mostly to companies that require physical checkups for their employees and to companies that specialize in recruiting workers to be employed overseas.

BUDGET

For this highly technical and capital intensive clinic to achieve maximum efficiency, it is necessary to have intrinsic controls over resources and services. The primary means by

*Source: Reprinted from C.L. Bautista, Meeting the Challenge of Cost Containment: A Case Study Using Variance Analysis, *Topics in Health Care Finance,* Vol. 21, No. 1, pp. 13–23, © 1994, Aspen Publishers, Inc.

which the clinic accomplishes this goal is by establishing and administering an annual operating budget. The budget serves as a tool to effectively manage and optimize the use of available resources and make wise choices among competing demands. This overall plan for the coordination of resources covers a defined period of time and is designed according to the assessed current and future market demands.

This statement of anticipated results may be expressed in financial terms (i.e., revenue and expense or capital budgets) or in nonfinancial terms (i.e., direct labor hours, materials, or production units). As such, having a budget annually assists the manager in formulating strategic, financial, operational, and clinical plans that systematize resource utilization and control.

At the end of each budget, periodic performance analysis is executed to recognize potential and developing problems and to take timely corrective actions as opportunities present themselves. The object of performance analysis is to identify cost variances to the budget and to minimize the efficiency cost in any given situation. The first step in the process is to compare the actual costs incurred in producing the services delivered for a particular time period with the budgeted values. The difference between these two values is called a variance. Should actual costs exceed or drastically fall below budgeted values, the manager then investigates the different factors that produced such variance. The sooner problems or opportunities are recognized, the sooner inefficiency costs are minimized. For this reason, it is imperative that each expense account be analyzed through the use of a series of variance reporting activities.

COST VARIANCE REPORTING

Variance reports identify and measure the factors that affect current performance levels.

The analysis procedure assists management in identifying differences due specifically to usage of resources, rates paid, and productivity of paid personnel. Productivity costs, for example, are analyzed in terms of actual labor costs per examination versus standard costs, or total costs per examination compared at different time periods.

Volume variances could stem from an increase or reduction in the number and strength of competitors, changes in a particular third party payer contract, or from failure to recognize the changing health care needs of the community it serves. Furthermore, volume changes could result from positive or negative outcomes of marketing efforts undertaken by the organization.

The common causes of labor efficiency variances include erroneous staffing, poor scheduling as evidenced by prolonged idle time or delays, inaccurate setting of standards with respect to the labor hours required for a given level of output, and/or unanticipated changes in the clinic's operation (i.e., breakdown of equipment, improved scheduling systems, automation changes, or changes in staffing skill levels).

The third variance factor is the labor or supply rate variance. Unforeseen changes in inflation may cause the rise or fall of wage or price increases unequal to planned levels. It may also result from personnel working a significant amount of unplanned overtime due to volume or operational pattern changes (i.e., rapid staff turnover resulting in incongruous staffing mix).

Separating variances into distinct categories and reporting these periodically hastens the identification of current and potential problem areas. Specific cost variance reports serve as the framework for determining possible causes of problems and objectively measuring the magnitude of the problem. It establishes a basis for trend analysis and facilitates the selection of effective and realistic solutions.

TOOL USED IN BUDGETING AND VARIANCE REPORTING

The clinic has invested in a Cost Management Information (CMI) system used to develop the annual budget. The system initially quantifies all resources used by the clinic throughout the previous year. This value is then adjusted for resource requirements based on anticipated future demands to produce the estimated resource requirements for the next year.

Each service provided to patients is described in terms of an output measure of work load. The resources used to produce each unit of output are then quantified in terms of staff, space, and supplies expenses. To properly allocate resources with reference to volume fluctuations, such cost components are further subdivided into variable and fixed costs. Moreover, expenses are classified into functional groupings that may be used in performing procedure costing and productivity monitoring.

Therefore, the CMI system assists the manager in collecting, analyzing, and incorporating into the budgeting process anticipated work load statistics, the number of full-time equivalent (FTE) staff, and the amount of supplies required to complete the job. In the following section, the 1992 budget and actual expense reports of the LRL Radiology Diagnostic Clinic are followed by an analysis that uses a series of variance reports to chart the clinic's past year performance.

COST ANALYSIS OF THE LRL RADIOLOGY DIAGNOSTIC CLINIC

In formulating the budget for 1992, the manager used the clinic's actual work load output and the volume and mix of patients served in 1991 and adjusted it for forecasted demand generated from environmental scanning activities. An estimated volume of 5,000 imaging procedures per month was expected for 1992. Based on this volume, the manager calculated the number of FTEs and the volume of supplies required to deliver this service. Expressed in dollar amounts, the budgeted costs for salaries and wages was $919,661.30, whereas that of supplies was $606,493.68. To analyze the clinic's performance for 1992, the actual volume or cost of resources consumed to produce the services delivered were compared with the established budget.

Exhibit 1 shows that the actual costs incurred for salaries and wages in 1992 exceeded the budgeted amounts by $35,288.35, or 4 percent, whereas the costs of supplies were less than expected by $9,234.27, or 2 percent. The specific factors that led to these results, however, cannot be determined by using this report. The report only provides a starting point for comparing the clinic's performance.

To get a more detailed look at the year's activity, it is necessary to generate the monthly status reports categorized by expense account. Exhibit 2 shows the clinic's 1992 expense report for the last 6 months of 1992 and budgeted and actual totals for the full year. This format isolates and provides a means to measure the impact that each variance factor plays in affecting performance.

The "budgeted per year" and "actual per year" columns of Exhibit 2 show that 1992 actual expenses exceeded budgeted values in salaries paid to the X-ray technicians, darkroom technicians, and radiologists, whereas actual expenses fell short of the budgeted value in the office aide category. Unfavorable variances are also seen in the categories of X-ray films, contrast media, other patient supplies, printing, housekeeping, and maintenance.

Exhibit 1 LRL Radiology Diagnostic Clinic

Annual Expense Report				
Period Ending December 31, 1992				
Description	**Budgeted**	**Actual**	**Variance**	**Percentage**
Salaries/wages	$919,661.30	$954,949.65	$(35,288.35)	(4.0%)
Supplies	606,493.68	597,259.41	9,234.27	2.0%
Total	$1,526,154.98	$1,552,209.06	$(26,054.08)	(2.0%)

The next step performed in this analysis is to focus more closely on specific months where major variances occurred and further analyze those factors that caused this change. Exhibit 3 focuses on August 1992 in particular. It shows that the budgeted salary for the six X-ray technicians was $20,088.00; however, the actual amount paid was $26,568.00, including overtime. The actual expense for X-ray films amounted to $16,767.09, but only $15,641.00 was budgeted, leading to a variance of $1,126.09.

An examination of the clinic's statistics for August 1992 (see Exhibit 4) reveals that a significant increase in the volume of imaging procedure occurred in that month. The actual volume of chest X-ray and mammography procedures exceeded the budgeted volumes by 638 and 225, respectively. This increase in volume may have accounted for the unbudgeted $6,480.00 in overtime pay received by the X-ray technicians, as well as the $1,126.09 applied to the purchase of X-ray films. This model also applies to variances seen in the salary paid to the radiologist and the darkroom technicians and to the supply variance costs. Consequently, the manager performed a series of variance analyses to identify and quantify the actual monthly expenses incurred according to the type and quantity of procedures delivered; the time requirement for completing these procedures; the current cost of materials, labor, and other cost components; and other possible factors that lead to changes in cost.

The reports shown in Exhibits 5 through 7 provide the detail for analyzing the volume, labor, and efficiency cost variances of the LRL Radiology Diagnostic Clinic. The labor costs for August 1992 are analyzed in greater detail in Exhibit 5, the Monthly Labor Rate Variance Report, which measures the difference between the standard labor rate and what was actually paid. Exhibit 6, the Monthly Labor Volume Variance Report, measures the difference between the labor hours consumed and the labor hours budgeted for the month's output level. Both reports compare what the staff was paid and what the staff was allotted to receive. The clinic manager uses such information to enhance her ability to monitor labor costs and to provide guidance for the direction and substance of future wage plans.

It can be seen from these reports that the X-ray technicians were paid an average rate of $13.06/hour in comparison to the original budget of $12.00/hour. Again, the variance was due to the staff working a significant amount of unanticipated overtime for this period. The budgeted hours totaled 279 for the month, whereas the actual hours earned amounted to 339.

The labor efficiency variance for X-ray technicians can be calculated by measuring the difference between the actual hours con-

Exhibit 2 Expense reports

Salary and Wage Expense Report
Variable Budget for Period Ending December 31, 1992

Code	Description	Standard rate	July	August	September	October
	Days		31.00	31.00	30.00	31.00
488	Manager	135.00	4,185.00	4,185.00	4,050.00	4,185.00
	15.00/hr*9hrs					
489	Accountant	126.00	3,206.00	3,906.00	3,780.00	3,906.00
	18.00/hr*7hrs					
467	Sys. Analyst	95.90	2,972.90	2,972.90	2,877.00	2,972.90
	13.70/hr*7hrs					
528	Office Aides	192.99	4,503.10	5,982.69	5,789.70	5,982.69
	9.19/hr*7hrs					
505	US Tech	168.00	5,208.00	5,208.00	5,040.00	5,208.00
	12.00/hr*7hrs					
	OT	18.00				
504	X-ray Tech	648.00	20,088.00	20,088.00	19,440.00	20,088.00
	12.00/hr*7hrs					
	OT	18.00	6,480.00	6,480.00		
514	Dkrm Tech	171.00	5,301.00	5,301.00	5,130.00	5,301.00
	9.50/hr*9hrs					
	OT	14.25	1,140.00	1,140.00		
507	Nurse Aides	189.00	5,859.00	5,859.00	5,670.00	5,859.00
	13.50/hr*7hrs					
	OT	20.25				
500	Radiologist	739.83	24,605.63	24,605.63	23,811.90	24,605.63
	35.23/hr*7hrs					
	OT	52.83	1,056.60	1,056.60		
	Salary/Wage		85,305.23	86,784.82	75,588.60	78,108.22

Supply Expense Report
Variable Budget for Period Ending December 31, 1992

Code	Description	Standard rate	July	August	September	October
116	X-ray Films	15,641.00	16,767.09	16,767.09	15,492.00	14,468.00
	553.66	28.25 (Rolls)				
126	Cont. Media	22,287.00	23,089.29	23,089.29	19,821.00	19,899.00
	394.46	56.50 (Bottles)				
144	Surg. Instr.	2,640.00	2,965.00	2,971.00	2,577.00	2,627.00
145	Other Supply	5,000.00	6,347.00	6,415.00	5,411.00	4,681.00
204	Printing	2,784.00	3,841.00	3,532.00	2,764.00	2,654.00
350	Housekeeping	347.00	415.00	462.00	254.00	199.00
205	Subscription	20.14	0.00	84.68	0.00	0.00
222	Maintenance	2,054.00	2,483.00	0.00	0.00	0.00
	Total		55,907.38	53,650.06	46,319.00	44,528.00
	Grand Total		141,212.61	140,434.88	121,907.60	122,636.22

November	December	OT	Budgeted per year	Actual per year	Variance	% Variance
30.00	31.00					
4,050.00	4,185.00		49,275.00	49,275.00	0.00	0.00
3,780.00	3,960.00		45,990.00	45,990.00	0.00	0.00
2,877.00	2,972.90		35,003.50	35,003.50	0.00	0.00
5,789.70	5,982.69		70,441.35	68,961.76	1,479.59	0.02
5,040.00	5,208.00		61,320.00	61,320.00	0.00	0.00
19,440.00	20,088.00		236,520.00	264,708.00	(28,188.00)	(0.12)
5,130.00	5,301.00	28,188.00	62,415.00	67,402.50	(4,987.50)	(0.08)
5,670.00	5,859.00	4,987.50	68,985.00	68,985.00	0.00	0.00
23,811.90	24,605.63		289,711.45	293,303.89	(3,592.44)	(0.01)
75,588.60	78,108.22	3,592.44 36,767.94	919,661.30	954,949.65	(35,288.35)	(0.04)

November	December	OT	Budgeted per year	Actual per year	Variance	% Variance
15,008.00	15,341.00		187,692.00	190,085.48	(2,393.48)	(0.01)
18,997.00	18,467.00		267,444.00	257,694.97	9,749.03	0.04
2,218.00	1,972.00		31,440.00	32,002.00	(562.00)	(0.02)
5,006.00	4,251.00		60,000.00	65,959.00	(5,959.00)	(0.10)
2,684.00	2,879.00		33,408.00	37,087.00	(3,679.00)	(0.11)
164.28	325.00		1,620.00	3,974.28	(2,354.28)	(1.45)
0.00	0.00		241.68	241.68	0.00	0.00
0.00	0.00		24,648.00	10,215.00	14,433.00	0.59
44,077.28	43,235.00		606,493.68	597,259.41	9,234.27	0.02
119,665.88	121,343.22		1,526,154.98	1,552,209.06	(26,054.08)	(0.02)

Exhibit 3 Variance report for the period August 1–31, 1992

Code	Description	Actual YTD	Budgeted YTD	Variance	% Variance	Monthly actual	Monthly budget	Variance	% Variance
	Days					31.00			
488	Manager	32,805.00	32,805.00	0.00	0.00	4,185.00	4,185.00	0.00	0.00
489	Accountant	30,618.00	30,618.00	0.00	0.00	3,906.00	3,906.00	0.00	0.00
467	Sys. Analyst	23,303.70	23,303.70	(0.00)	(0.00)	2,972.90	2,972.90	(0.00)	(0.00)
528	Office Aides	45,416.98	46,911.15	1,494.17	0.03	5,982.69	5,982.69	0.00	0.00
505	US Tech	40,824.00	40,824.00	0.00	0.00	5,208.00	5,208.00	0.00	0.00
	Overtime								
504	X-ray Tech	185,652.00	157,464.00	(28,188.00)	(0.18)	20,088.00	20,088.00	0.00	0.00
	Overtime					6,480.00		(6,480.00)	
514	Dkrm.Tech	46,540.50	41,553.00	(4,987.50)	(0.12)	5,301.00	5,301.00	0.00	0.00
	Overtime					1,140.00		(1,140.00)	
507	Nurse Aides	45,927.00	45,927.00	0.00	0.00	5,859.00	5,859.00	0.00	0.00
	Overtime								
500	Radiologist	196,468.83	192,876.39	(3,592.44)	(0.02)	24,605.63	24,605.63	0.00	0.00
	Overtime					1,056.60		(1,056.60)	
	Salary/Wage	647,556.01	612,282.24	(35,273.77)	(0.06)	86,784.82	78,108.22	(8,676.60)	(0.11)

Code	Description	Actual YTD	Budgeted YTD	Variance	% Variance	Monthly actual	Monthly budget	Variance	% Variance
116	X-Ray Films	129,776.48	125,128.00	(4,648.48)	(0.04)	16,767.09	15,641.00	(1,126.09)	(0.07)
126	Cont. Media	180,510.97	178,296.00	(2,214.97)	(0.01)	23,089.29	22,287.00	(802.29)	(0.04)
144	Surg. Instr	22,608.00	21,120.00	(1,488.00)	(0.07)	2,971.00	2,640.00	(331.00)	(0.13)
145	Other Supply	46,610.00	40,000.00	(6,610.00)	(0.17)	6,415.00	5,000.00	(1,415.00)	(0.28)
204	Printing	26,106.00	22,272.00	(3,834.00)	(0.17)	3,861.00	2,784.00	(1,077.00)	(0.39)
350	Housekeeping	3,032.00	2,776.00	(256.00)	(0.09)	462.00	347.00	(115.00)	(0.33)
205	Subscriptions	241.68	161.12	(80.56)	(0.50)	84.68	20.14	(64.54)	(3.20)
222	Maintenance	10,215.00	16,432.00	6,217.00	0.38	0.00	2,054.00	2054.00	1.00
	Total	419,100.13	406,185.12	(12,915.01)	(0.03)	53,650.06	50,773.14	(2,876.92)	(0.06)
	Grand Total	1,066,656.14	1,018,467.36	(48,188.78)	(0.05)	140,434.88	128,881.36	(11,553.52)	(0.09)

sumed to produce the given level of output with the standard labor hours estimated for the same level of output. As seen in Exhibit 7, the standard hours for producing 5,067 images for the six X-ray technicians was 212. This figure is based on the industry-wide statistical standard. However, the actual hours it took the six technicians to produce the same number of images was 249. Therefore, it took the six technicians 37 hours more to produce the same volume of work load output.

Based on the findings, the decline in efficiency was a result of unanticipated changes in the department's production process. Due to an unforeseen increase in volume, the clinic's scheduling pattern was disrupted. This resulted in delays in client processing. Furthermore, because of the large volumes, the current staff could not handle the load and became overburdened, which contributed to further production delays.

Reporting the labor efficiency levels by skill level leads to a better understanding and analysis of the clinic's productivity and efficiency and serves as a signal to update procedure standards if inconsistent or unrealistic values are attained. This information can be incorporated into a flexible budget to analyze the budget resources required for an actual level of activity.

In reviewing and analyzing the events that transpired in 1992, the staff discovered that

Exhibit 4 Radiology diagnostic clinic statistics for the month of August 1992

Description	Budget	Actual	Variance
Chest	3,055	3,693	(638)
Abdominal	95	20	75
GI/Esophagus	85	35	50
Gall Bladder	15	15	0
B. Enema	44	40	4
I.V.P.	12	10	2
Extremities	650	412	238
Skull	31	0	31
Spine	250	126	124
Mammogram	450	675	(225)
Other	0	0	0
Subtotal	4,687	5,026	(339)
Ultrasound:			
Breast	12	20	(8)
Gall Bladder	16	24	(8)
Renal	10	15	(5)
Liver	42	35	7
Pelvis	7	14	(7)
Ob/Gyn	225	235	(10)
Pancreas	6	4	2
Spleen	7	5	2
Other	0	0	0
Subtotal	325	352	(27)
Grand Total	5,012	5,378	(366)

the unanticipated increase in volume resulted from the January 1992 closure of a competitor's clinic. Not only did this event reduce competition for the LRL Radiology, but it also resulted in a positive change in the physician and staff complement. In June 1992, the clinic hired a radiologist who was previously employed at the other facility. This physician replaced a radiologist who left the clinic to take a fellowship in London. This change further increased the monthly output.

No price or salary changes occurred during that period, thereby eliminating this variable as a cause for the variance. Apparently, the difference in the office aides' yearly expense is due to the resignation of one of the office aides in July 1992. This left the clinic with two full-time aides for 20 days until the third person was replaced by an aide who had been previously employed at the competitor's office. The analysis confirmed an assumption that the unanticipated volume resulted from underestimated overtime and supplies costs rather than price or wage increases.

RECOMMENDATIONS

The manager of the clinic monitored cost expenses using an annual budget that estimated the resource requirements for a given period of time, based on a static volume of demand and then compared it with the actual cost for the actual output attained. Although this method provided the clinic with sufficient guidelines to monitor resource utilization and productivity, it did not provide enough detail to ascertain what particular factor, or factors, led to the resulting variance.

In this particular case study, the supplies variance was determined to be the result of increased cost incurred. However, using this method, the office manager was unable to point out the degree to which the price of supplies affected the overall cost or to what degree the volume of supplies used per procedure deviated from the estimated values.

The clinic will benefit from applying flexible budgeting techniques in the succeeding years to develop a more accurate determination of cost calculations. Flexible budgeting reflects expected revenues and expenses at various levels of patient utilization. It recognizes the difficulty of establishing a single optimum level of achievement and provides a tool for controlling costs at various levels.

To flex the budget, the original budgeted amount must be adjusted to reflect the actual volume of procedures performed during the budget period. This new value, called the flexible budget, is then subtracted from the original budget to reflect the volume variance. The resulting volume variance accounts

Exhibit 5 Monthly labor rate variance analysis report

					Report period: August 1–31, 1992			
Code	Description	Standard rate per staff	Actual rate per staff	Actual hours	Actual hrs. actual rate	Actual hrs. standard rate	Labor rate variance	% Variance
505	US Tech	12.00	12.00	217	2,604.00	2,604.00	0.00	0.00
504	X-ray Tech	12.00	13.06	339	4,427.34	4,068.00	(359.34)	(0.09)
514	Dkrm Tech	9.50	10.10	319	3,221.90	3,030.50	(191.40)	(0.06)

Exhibit 6 Monthly labor volume variance analysis report

					Report period: August 1–31, 1992			
Code	Description	Standard rate per staff	Hours earned	Hours budgeted	Earned hrs. standard rate	Budgeted hrs. standard rate	Labor volume variance	% Variance
505	US Tech	12.00	279	279	3,348.00	3,348.00	(0.00)	0.00
504	X-ray Tech	12.00	339	279	4,068.00	3,348.00	(720.00)	(0.22)
514	Dkrm Tech	9.50	319	279	3,030.50	2,650.50	(380.00)	(0.14)

Exhibit 7 Labor efficiency variance report

				Report period: August 1–31, 1992		
Code	Description	Standard wage rate	Actual hours	Earned hours	Actual hrs. standard rate	Earned hrs. standard rate	Efficiency variance
504	X-ray Tech	$12.00	212	249	2,544.00	2,988.00	(444.00)
514	Dkrm Tech	$9.50	200	229	1,900.00	2,175.50	(275.50)

Exhibit 8 Monthly supply variance report

				Report period: August 1–31, 1992			
Code	Description	Actual expense	Flexed expense	Budgeted expense	Rate variance	Volume variance	Total variance	% Variance
116	X-Ray Film	16,767.09	16,609.80	15,641.00	(157.29)	(968.80)	(1,126.09)	(0.07)
126	Cont. Media	23,089.29	22,878.68	22,287.00	(210.61)	(591.68)	(802.29)	(0.04)

for the degree of variance caused by an unanticipated change in work load.

Exhibit 8, the Monthly Supply Variance Report, shows how flexible budgeting techniques are used. The variable portions of the budgeted expense for supplies and purchased services have been adjusted to reflect the change in volume and are labeled "Flexed Expense." The chart shows that the additional costs incurred resulted from an increase in volume and not from a rise in the price of supplies or a rise in the inefficient use of supplies. If the manager had used this technique in the past, then she could have allotted more resources during those peak months.

In addition to cost-saving tools such as the annual budget and variance reports, corrective action in the form of adjusting staffing levels, cross-training of staff, enhancing automation, improving production techniques, and improving scheduling patterns may be incorporated into the budget planning process to eliminate inefficiencies.

To provide the skills needed now and in the future, cross-training of staff members will be critical. Cross-training increases staff flexibility and adaptability in addressing unanticipated situations. By being able to adjust staffing levels when trends are noticed, the manager will be able to more efficiently mix staffing skill levels to produce the optimal outcome at less cost.

Finally, recent advances in information systems have provided managers with a more effective way of streamlining, monitoring, and expediting the delivery of products and services through automating the process of generating radiology reports and films. This includes accepting orders, scheduling patients to rooms, assigning resources and staff to patients, assigning codes to cases, performing quality assurance functions, tracking patients and film, monitoring inventory, clarifying billing, and tracking who did what and when within the clinic.

Therefore, such systems increase the integration of clinical and operational activities. They provide the clinic with a means of achieving marked improvements in organizational restructuring, work load balancing, work force balancing, reducing costs, and delivering service as a result of more accurate and timely information collection and retrieval.

Trend analysis may be used to determine the progress of staffing changes that result from focused productivity studies. By isolating and identifying these controlled variables and comparing them with the standards, an objective evaluation necessity and cost-effectiveness is obtained.

Through the use of budgeting techniques such as flexible budgeting and various management information systems, the clinic manager will be able to monitor resource consumption and productivity levels more closely. With this information at hand, problem areas will be found rapidly, and more effective solutions will be implemented.

BIBLIOGRAPHY

Baptist, A.J. "A General Approach to Costing Procedures in Ancillary Departments." *Topics in Health Care Financing* 13, no. 4 (1987): 32–47.

Bolster, C.J., and Bibion, R. "Linkages Between Cost Management and Productivity." *Topics in Health Care Financing* 13, no. 4 (1987): 67–75.

Finkler, S.A. *Budgeting for Nurse Managers.* 2nd ed. Philadelphia, Pa.: W.B. Saunders, 1992.

Finkler, S.A. "Flexible Budget Variance Analysis Extended to Patient Activity and DRGs." *Health Care Management Review* 10, no. 4 (1985): 21–34.

Horngren, C.T., and Foster, G. *Cost Accounting: A Managerial Emphasis*, 6th ed. Englewood Cliffs, N.J.: Prentice Hall, 1987.

Lopez, L.R., and Ignacio, V. Personal interview. Manila, the Philippines, 2 September 1993.

Nackel, J., Kis, G., and Fenaroli, P. "Managing with Cost Information." In *Cost Management for Hospitals*. Gaithersburg, Md.: Aspen Publishers, 1987.

PART V

Mini-Case Studies

CHAPTER 16

Mini-Case Study 1:
Using Financial Ratios and
Interpreting Credit Analysis in
Hospitals and Nursing Homes

Hospital Finance*

Mark J. Herman

Today, the health care industry, and more specifically, the hospital segment, face unprecedented change. Rapidly evolving regulatory and reimbursement policies, continued cost pressures, increased competition, an expanding managed care presence, and a more sophisticated, demanding, and knowledgeable purchasing marketplace combine to create an environment in which only the financially strong and managerially adept will survive. Consequently, sorting out the winners from the losers is as much a matter of strategy assessment as it is pure financial analysis. The following presents an overview of key focus areas for scrutiny when lending to the hospital segment.

TAX STATUS

The tax status of a hospital can be either a 501(c)(3) not-for-profit or a taxable C-Corporation. The status elected will have numerous implications on the strategic financial management of the organization. Table 1 summarizes the major operating differences.

REGULATORY ENVIRONMENT

Hospital regulations are burdensome and complex. Licensing, revenue reimbursement, and reporting all play a material role in a hospital's long-term viability. Hospitals are licensed in their respective state(s) of operation and are accredited by the Joint Commission on Accreditation of Healthcare Organizations (Joint Commission). Collectively, this process defines and oversees the activities of hospital operations.

Hospital revenue is typically dominated by Medicare (a federal program for patients 65 years or older) and Medicaid (a state-administered and partially federally funded program for the poor). These government programs provide the majority of payments to the providers via a prospective diagnosis-related group (DRG) payment system, whereby a fixed amount of revenue is received per DRG case regardless of the costs incurred. A cost report is submitted annually to Medicare and Medicaid for revenue reimbursement audit and settlement of overpayments or underpayments.

Capital expenditures above a maximum predetermined threshold are regulated in many states and require approval of a certificate of need. Antifraud, antitrust, Stark II (fraudulent referrals), and utilization reviews are just a few of the additional regulatory re-

*Source: Reprinted from M.J. Herman, Hospital Finance, *Journal of Health Care Finance,* Vol. 24, No. 4, pp. 22–26, © 1998, Aspen Publishers, Inc.

Table 1 The Major Operating Differences between a Hospital with a 501(c)(3) Not-for-Profit Tax Status and a Hospital with a Taxable C-Corporation Tax Status

	501(c)(3)	*C-Corp.*
Taxes		
Income (federal, state, local)	No	Yes
Property	No	Yes
Sales	No	Yes
Capital access		
Debt	Tax exempt	Taxable
Equity	No	Yes
Charity care	All patients regardless of ability to pay	Controllable patient selection

quirements. Failure to comply can, in its most serious state, suspend revenue reimbursement and/or cost the provider its license to operate.

MANAGEMENT

In order to lead and compete effectively in today's complex health care marketplace, a management team must possess numerous skills. These should include demonstrated competencies in financial and cost management, physician relations, managed care contracting, staff negotiations, legal and regulatory compliance, information technology, and risk and change management. The ability to shape and transform a vision founded on a true understanding of macro- and microenvironmental factors will enhance the survival of any entity. Get to know the management of your borrower as intimately as possible. It is this collective human resource that will create organizational success or, conversely, become its downfall.

COMPETITIVE ENVIRONMENT

The key question to ask in your competitive analysis is "Does your borrower possess the ability to differentiate itself and sustain an advantage over time to allow it to be a long-term industry survivor?" To partially answer this question, a lender needs to answer the following 10 questions:

1. What differentiates the borrower from its competitors? (Product offerings, geographic delivery, low cost products, etc.)
2. Does the borrower have a formal defined strategic plan?
3. What primary and secondary market share is held by the borrower?
4. What is the payer mix in the borrower's defined target market?
5. What percentage of revenues is managed care contracts? What are the trends? How much financial risk is held by the borrower?
6. What insurance coverages exist to mitigate risk?
7. Is medical technology current and will future technology investments be adequate to sustain leading edge quality outcomes?
8. Are information systems adequate to report reliable, timely, and accurate quality data, cost data, and useful management financial information? Does the existing system contain ad-

equate expansion capability? Is the borrower adequately addressing the millennium 2000 issue?

9. Does management demonstrate an aptitude and willingness to provide regular, meaningful dialogue with its financial suppliers?

10. Does the borrower have adequate financial capacity to meet all necessary ongoing capital requirements?

FINANCIAL ANALYSIS

When analyzing the financial condition of a hospital, three important areas to review are the hospital's cash flow, balance sheet liquidity, and leverage. These focal points should be viewed in combination with general operational, balance sheet trends, and important utilization statistics.

CASH FLOW

Analysis of a hospital's cash flow is very important since internal cash flow generation provides the funds necessary to service debt and make capital expenditures and/or acquisitions.

Cash flow generation ability is measured by the industry using the debt service coverage ratio (DSCR). The DSCR is often the primary financial covenant in the hospital's Master Trust Indenture and debt or loan agreements with other financing sources such as banks and insurance companies. The DSCR is calculated by taking the sum of the hospital's increase in net assets (net income), depreciation, interest, and any noncash charges and extraordinary items. The sum of these items becomes the numerator of the calculation known as cash flow available for debt service. The denominator of the calculation is composed of the principal and interest payments on all debt obligations of the hospi-

tal to include long-term debt from bond issues, bank term loans and lines of credit, capital leases, and any contingent debt.

This ratio measures the number of times a hospital's debt service requirements could be met from existing cash flow and helps to determine its ability to add or increase debt financing. A higher DSCR generally means a stronger ability to cover debt service obligations, and a greater likelihood of having additional cash flow left over to cover capital expenditures. The minimum DSCR acceptable to most lenders is a range of 1.25–1.40 times; however, financing sources prefer to see DSCRs substantially higher, in the 2.0–3.5 times range. It is also important to assess the ongoing maintenance capital expenditures of the hospital and whether internal cash flow generation will be sufficient to cover those expenditures, or whether borrowing or taking on additional debt will be necessary.

LIQUIDITY

The analysis of the hospital's balance sheet liquidity is very important as unrestricted liquidity can provide cushion should internal cash flow generation be tight, can cover unforeseen needs for cash, and can provide internal funding for capital expenditures and acquisitions.

Balance sheet liquidity is measured using the days cash on hand (DCOH) ratio, which indicates the number of days that a hospital could cover its operating expenses (excluding depreciation and interest) with its unrestricted cash and investments if no future revenues were to be received. DCOH is measured by taking the amount of unrestricted cash and investments on the balance sheet, both current and long-term, and multiplying the result by the number of days in the measurement period (365 days for a full year), this product being the numerator of the ratio.

The denominator is the operating expenses for the period being measured, excluding bad debt expense, interest expense, and depreciation expense.

This ratio yields the number of days' cash a hospital has on hand. This number can vary greatly from one state to another depending on its operating environment, the amount of regulation, managed care penetration, and the hospital's tax status. An average number of DCOH in New York for a nonprofit hospital would be 30 days versus 100 days in Michigan. For-profit hospitals would have significantly lower DCOH ratios, some approaching zero if all of the hospital's cash is held at the parent company level. As a general rule, DCOH of less than 60 days for a nonprofit would be of concern depending upon the intricacies of the state in which the hospital operates. Sources of unrestricted liquidity would be short-term unrestricted cash and investments, marketable securities, funded depreciation (found in assets whose use is limited in noncurrent assets), and other sources of unrestricted balance sheet cash such as significant overfunding of a malpractice fund. Many hospitals across the country have built up large cash reserves equal to or greater than the amount of debt on the balance sheet. Nonprofit hospitals typically borrow at attractive tax-exempt rates rather than use internally generated cash to pay for capital expenditures and then arbitrage their large cash reserves on the balance sheet at higher taxable rates.

LEVERAGE

Leverage is most commonly measured using the total liabilities/unrestricted net assets ratio, which reflects the extent to which a hospital relies on debt to finance its balance sheet assets and often serves as an indicator of the hospital's capital structure. This ratio can also indicate the ability to borrow additional long-term funds. It is calculated by dividing total liabilities by unrestricted net assets (fund balances). The primary source of asset financing for nonprofit hospitals is long-term tax-exempt bond debt, while for-profit hospitals utilize both equity offerings and long-term taxable bond debt. The capital structures of nonprofit and for-profit hospitals vary greatly. Nonprofit hospitals are generally more conservative than their for-profit competitors and have a lower leverage ratio—under 1.5:1.0. Larger hospital systems and teaching tertiary nonprofits have higher leverage ratios of up to 2.0:1.0, a function of the need to continually invest in the latest high technology equipment.

•   •   •

Lending to the hospital segment has never been more difficult. After the loan is made, the job has barely begun. Keeping apprised of events and trends in health care and understanding their effects on each of your customers and prospects requires vigilance. Candid discussions regarding vision, strategies, and tactics are mandatory in order for you to formulate an opinion as to the viability of the organization. Continuous communications with key management, reviewing and monitoring the progress of their plans, and frequent tracking of the key financial ratios are the best available means to validate your decision.

Credit Analysis of a Skilled Nursing Facility*

Seth Siegel

CASE STUDY: XYZ

To illustrate the fundamental issues related to analyzing a non-profit skilled nursing facility credit, a case study of a hypothetical skilled nursing facility, XYZ,[1] has been created. To facilitate this analysis, XYZ's ratios have been calculated and compared to the Fitch IBCA non-profit skilled nursing medians. It is important to recognize that while this analysis focuses on the financial strengths and weaknesses of XYZ, other factors that are briefly mentioned in the "Background of XYZ," such as management and board experience, facility location, and competitive pressures, are equally important in evaluating its overall strength. Table 1 provides a summary of XYZ's financial statements.

Background of XYZ

XYZ is a non-profit skilled nursing facility constructed in 1990. It consists of 160 skilled nursing beds. XYZ has benefitted from minimal competition and an average occupancy exceeding 95% during the last three years. The facility's management is experienced and competent. Its change in unrestricted assets has shown steady, marked improvement. Its board of directors has been effective in directing the facility's goals.

XYZ, looking to reduce its interest expense, now wishes to refund its outstanding $9,450,000 of Series 1990 unrated tax-exempt bonds, originally issued for the construction of the facility.

Three factors influencing the economic feasibility of XYZ's refunding are: 1) the current interest rate environment compared to the interest rate environment in 1990, 2) the optional redemption provisions of the Series 1990 bonds, and 3) the ability of XYZ to obtain a stand-alone rating. Obviously, lower interest rates, flexible redemption provisions, and a conversion of the Series 1990 bonds from unrated to rated all increase the likelihood of an economically feasible refunding. For this analysis, the impact of interest rates and the Series 1990 bond's optional redemption provisions are not considered; the focus of this analysis will be on XYZ's ability to obtain a rating.

Analysis of XYZ

In order for a credit analysis to be meaningful, it is necessary to review at least two years of a facility's operating history. Two

*Source: Reprinted from S. Siegel, Credit Analysis of a Skilled Nursing Facility, *Journal of Health Care Finance,* Vol. 26, No. 2 (in press), © 1999, Aspen Publishers, Inc.

Table 1 XYZ's Financial Statements

Statement Of Changes In Unrestricted Net Assets (Income Statement) (000's)		
	1997	*1998*
OPERATING REVENUES		
Operating Revenue	$6,540	$6,808
Other Operating Revenue	419	323
Total Operating Revenue	**6,959**	**7,131**
OPERATING EXPENSES		
Operations	5,372	5,465
Depreciation and Amortization	578	590
Interest	917	905
Total Operating Expenses	**6,867**	**6,960**
Operating Income	92	171
NON-OPERATING REVENUES		
Contributions	23	25
Gain on Sale of Assets	51	27
Unrealized Gain on Securities	23	28
Change in Unrestricted Net Assets	**189**	**251**

Statement Of Financial Position (Balance Sheet) (000's)		
	1997	*1998*
ASSETS		
Cash and Investments— Unrestricted	$1,895	$2,094
Cash and Investments— Restricted	2,039	2,326
Accounts Receivable	493	483
Third-Party Settlements, Est.	242	428
Property, Plant & Equipment, Net	5,279	4,693
Debt Issuance Costs, Net	304	285
Other Assets	138	147
Total Assets	**$10,390**	**$10,456**
LIABILITIES		
Current Liabilities	$1,019	$1,029
Long-Term Debt	9,600	9,450
Residents' Deposits	71	79
Total Liabilities	10,690	10,029
Unrestricted Net Assets	(300)	(102)
Total Liabilities and Net Assets	**$10,390**	**$10,456**

years of predictable performance form the basis of a trend. If there is significant disparity between years, further analysis may be required. If, however, ratios are consistent among years, it is acceptable to focus on just the most recent year. XYZ's ratios are consistent; therefore, unless noted, our analysis centers on its most recent fiscal year, 1998. XYZ's financial ratios are summarized and compared to the Fitch IBCA medians in Table 2.

Profitability

XYZ demonstrates considerable operating strengths. Its Operating Margin Ratio of 2.4% and Total Excess Margin of 3.4% exceed Fitch IBCA medians.

XYZ's operating strength can be attributed to a number of factors. First, it has maintained an adequate pricing structure, adjusting its nursing fees to annually outpace rising nursing expenses.

Second, its nursing payor mix has remained very favorable: 50% private pay, 15% Medicare, 35% Medicaid. (Note: A higher percentage of private pay is desirable. The nursing industry average is 34% Private Pay, 58% Medicaid, and 8% Medicare and other.)[2]

Third, XYZ's investments have benefitted from the bull market of the 1990's. Its investment income, included in operating revenue,

Table 2 Ratio Calculations and XYZ versus Fitch IBCA Medians

Ratios	Ratio Calculations	Fitch IBCA Combined Medians	Facility XYZ	
			1997	1998
Profitability Ratios				
Operating Margin (%)	$\dfrac{\text{Operating Income (Loss)}}{\text{Total Operating Revenues}}$	1.7%	1.3%	2.4%
Total Excess Margin (%)	$\dfrac{\text{Change in Unrestricted Net Assets}}{\text{Total Revenues and Non-Operating Gains (Losses)}}$	2.8%	2.7%	3.4%
Operating Ratio (%)	$\dfrac{\text{Cash Operating Expenses}}{\text{Cash Operating Revenues}}$	93%	90.4%	89.3%
Capital Structure and Cash Flow Ratios				
Debt Service Coverage Ratio (x)	$\dfrac{\text{Change in Unrestricted Net Assets Plus Interest, Depreciation, Amortization}}{\text{Maximum Annual Debt Service*}}$	2.3	1.60	1.66
Debt to Capitalization (%)	$\dfrac{\text{Long-Term Debt, Less Current Portion}}{\text{Long-Term Debt, Less Current Portion Plus Unrestricted Net Assets}}$	47%	103.2	101.1%
Debt Service as a % of Total Revenue and Non Operating Gains (Losses) (%)	$\dfrac{\text{Maximum Annual Debt Service}}{\text{Total Revenues and Non-Operating Gains (Losses)}}$	6.8%	14.6%	14.1%
Liquidity Ratios				
Days Cash on Hand	$\dfrac{\text{Unrestricted Cash and Investments, Less Refundable Deposits}}{\text{Cash Operating Expenses/365}}$	107	110	120
Cushion Ratio (x)	$\dfrac{\text{Unrestricted Cash and Investments}}{\text{Maximum Annual Debt Service}}$	5.5	1.8	2.0

*XYZ's Maximum Annual Debt Service is assumed to be $1,035,000 for 1997 and 1998.

has consistently generated more than a 15% return.

XYZ's Operating Ratio at 89.3% is stronger than the Fitch IBCA (93.0%) median. XYZ's operating ratio for 1998 improved .9% over 1997. If this trend continues in 1999, its Operating Ratio will be a powerful indicator of the facility's ability to generate cash flow.

Capital Structure

XYZ's Capital Structure ratios present the weakest side of its financial picture. Its Debt Service Coverage Ratio of 1.66 falls significantly below the Fitch IBCA median (2.3). Such a ratio is acceptable for XYZ, however, because while it has a relatively high annual debt burden, its continues to generate enough cash flow not only to cover its debt but also to add to its cash balances. If XYZ's Debt Service Coverage Ratio ever fell below 1.20, analysts would have cause for concern.

XYZ's Debt to Capital Ratio of 101.1% is its weakest ratio. Fitch IBCA's median is 47%. Its negative fund balance is responsible for its high Debt to Capital Ratio. A negative trend in fund balance can be a sign that a facility is losing money. While XYZ has a negative fund balance—it incurred some planned losses for the first three years of operations (until occupancy was stabilized) and then booked two extraordinary losses—its fund balance has been improving and is scheduled to turn positive by the end of 1999.

Compared to the Fitch IBCA median (6.8%), XYZ's Debt Service as a Percentage of Total Revenue and Non-Operating Gains ratio of 14.1% is high. The reason for its high Debt Service as a Percentage of Total Revenue and Non-Operating Gains is XYZ's $9,450,000 of outstanding Series 1990 bonds. The Series 1999 refunding combined with strong operating performance will improve this ratio. This ratio should be reevaluated if and when XYZ explores raising additional capital for improvements or expansion.

Cash Position

XYZ's unrestricted cash has grown steadily since the facility began operations, averaging 2–10% annually. Unrestricted cash increased 10.5% from 1997 to 1998. In addition to healthy profit margins, because of the efforts of its fund-raising staff and volunteers, XYZ has been the beneficiary of some restricted and unrestricted contributions. These factors have placed XYZ in a strong cash position. Its Days Cash on Hand Ratio of 120 is respectable. It well exceeds the Fitch IBCA median (107).

While XYZ's Cushion Ratio of 2.0 is below Fitch IBCA's median of 5.5, its Cushion Ratio is not a concern. Taking into consideration that XYZ is refunding its Series 1990 bonds—with the intent of obtaining lower interest rates, and in turn, lowering its annual debt service payments—its cushion ratio will improve in 1999.

Results of XYZ Credit Analysis

When comparing XYZ to the Fitch IBCA medians, we recognize its many strengths and few weaknesses. Its operations exhibit a positive trend that will continue to add to its already healthy cash balances. And while XYZ's capital structure ratios depict a facility faced with the challenges of retiring debt and minimizing the impact of start-up losses, there is little cause for further inspection; its continued operating strength, stern monitorization of its patient mix, and proposed refinancing will do much to ameliorate these weaknesses. Facility XYZ will likely receive an investment grade rating.

NOTES

1. XYZ facility was created for purposes of this case study only; any resemblance of XYZ to another skilled nursing facility is coincidental.

2. SMG Marketing Group, 1993.

Credit Analysis of Nonprofit Continuing Care Retirement Communities*

Seth Siegel

INTRODUCTION

A burgeoning elderly population coupled with increased demand for a continuum of care for the elderly has spurred unprecedented growth among nonprofit continuing care retirement communities (CCRCs). In 1996, 219 facilities were financed with tax-exempt bonds, a 91 percent increase from the 20 financed in 1980. Between 1995 and 1996 alone, tax-exempt financing volume for nonprofit CCRCs increased nearly 25 percent.[1] And this growth, to the extent determined by demographics, is expected to continue. In this decade alone, the population over 65 and 85 will grow 13 percent and 48 percent, respectively.[2]

The exceptional growth of CCRCs has piqued the interest of the financial community. Amidst an ever-changing financial and regulatory environment, credit analysts are developing novel analytical tools and methodologies for evaluating CCRCs' financial strengths and weaknesses. This article discusses some of these prevailing tools and methodologies, provides a case study of a facility trying to obtain a stand-alone investment grade rating, and finishes with a review of recent changes in accounting standards and their impact on CCRC credit analysis.

The rating agencies

Three rating agencies provide ratings for CCRCs: Fitch Investors Service, Standard and Poor's Corporation, and Moody's Investors Service. Of the three rating agencies, Fitch has been the most active. It has issued 39 stand-alone and system ratings since 1989, when it published its rating guidelines for CCRCs. Standard and Poor's has issued 28 stand-alone and system ratings since it released its rating guidelines in 1992. And Moody's, which reentered the CCRC rating business in 1996, has issued four.[3]

Benchmarking studies

The American Association of Homes and Services for the Aging (AAHSA) and Fitch publish ratio reports that credit analysts use to benchmark CCRCs. AAHSA's publication, *Financial Ratios and Trend Analysis of CCAC Accredited Communities,* provides quartiles of 12 key ratios for single- and multisite Continuing Care Accreditation

*Source: Reprinted from S. Siegel, Credit Analysis of Nonprofit Continuing Care Retirement Communities, *Journal of Health Care Finance,* Vol. 24, No. 4, pp. 51–60, © 1998, Aspen Publishers, Inc.

Commission (CCAC) accredited facilities.[4,5]

Fitch's publication, *Health Care Financial Ratio Medians,* provides, by rating category (from lowest to highest: BB, BBB, and A), medians for the 25 CCRCs it has issued stand-alone ratings (e.g., no third party guarantee or credit enhancement).[6] Fitch also provides a median that combines its three rating categories. The CCAC medians for single-site facilities and the Fitch combined medians are shown in Table 1.

FINANCIAL RATIOS

In evaluating the financial strength of a CCRC, credit analysts focus on a combination of ratios. This article focuses on 10 ratios that provide the nucleus of a credit profile. The evaluation of one ratio cannot provide an accurate financial picture of a CCRC. Thus, no ratio should be viewed in isolation.

Absent in this analysis are the standard current and quick ratios. Because of the idiosyncracies of CCRC accounting, these ratios provide little meaning. When a facility issues debt, a trust indenture can impose restrictions on its cash balances. These restricted cash balances (e.g., a debt-service reserve fund or minimum liquid reserve requirement) are often classified as long term. This classification understates current assets in relation to current liabilities.

Another idiosyncracy of CCRC accounting is the amortization of entrance fees to operating revenue. Fitch, in its *Rating Guidelines for Nonprofit Continuing Care Retirement Communities,* describes this process:

> ...the actual cash a resident pays as an [entrance] fee is capitalized and then "earned" by the CCRC over the resident's life expectancy. No

"revenue" is recognized by the mere receipt of cash. Therefore, the total cash received for any given period bypasses the statement of revenues and expenses and, instead, appears on the cash flow statement. Revenue from [entrance] fees is recognized in the revenue and expense statement through an amortization process. In theory, this concept can be likened to the accounting treatment of depreciation expense.[7(p.11)]

This accounting treatment emphasizes a facility's reliance on revenues from entrance fees to cover operating expenses. The following ratios are adjusted to reflect this emphasis. Table 1 describes the calculation of the profitability, capital structure, and liquidity ratios.

Profitability ratios

Profitability ratios measure a CCRC's excess or deficiency of revenues over expenses. The three most widely used profitability ratios are the operating margin ratio, the total excess margin ratio, and the operating ratio.

The operating margin ratio indicates the excess of operating revenues after operating expenses have been covered. For this ratio, investment income is included as a source of revenue and contributions are excluded. (Revenue sources not integral to operations, such as gains and losses from disposition of assets, are excluded.) A ratio exceeding 0.00 percent is desirable.

Through the inclusion of nonoperating revenues, the total excess margin ratio provides a broader picture of profitability than the operating margin ratio. Extraordinary items and accounting changes are excluded. The typical

Table 1. Ratio Calculations and XYZ Versus Fitch and CCAC Medians

Ratios	Ratio calculations	Fitch combined medians	CCAC Single-site medians	Facility XYZ 1995	Facility XYZ 1996
Profitability ratios					
Operating margin (%)	Operating income (loss) / Total operating revenues	1.5%	1.0%	0.3%	2.8%
Total excess margin (%)	Change in unrestricted net assets / Total revenues and nonoperating gains (losses)	3.2%	4.5%	7.0%	6.4%
Operating ratio (%)	Cash operating expenses / Cash operating revenues	100.0%	102.7%	106.7%	103.7%
Capital structure and cash flow ratios					
Debt-service coverage ratio-unadjusted (x)	Change in unrestricted net assets plus interest, depreciation, amortization, less amortization of entrance fees, plus net entrance fees collected* / Maximum annual debt-service	2.0	2.32	1.60	1.65
Debt-service coverage ratio-adjusted (x)	Change in unrestricted net assets plus interest, depreciation, amortization, less amortization of entrance fees / Maximum annual debt-service	1.1	0.73	0.73	0.78
Unrestricted cash to debt (%)	Unrestricted cash and investments / Long-term debt, less current portion	N/A	46%	41%	42%
Debt to capitalization	Long-term debt, less current portion / Long-term debt, less current portion plus unrestricted net assets	64%	71%	130%	127%
Debt-service as a % of total revenue and nonoperating gains (losses) (%)	Maximum annual debt-service / Total revenues and nonoperating gains (losses)	11%	9%	34%	33%
Liquidity ratios					
Days cash on hand	Unrestricted cash and investments, less refundable deposits / Cash operating expenses/365	241	182	683	665
Cushion ratio (x)	Unrestricted cash and investments / Maximum annual debt-service	5.5	n/a	4.4	4.5

* Net entrance fees collected is a cash flow item, and is not presented in Tables 1 or 2. XYZ's net entrance fees collected are assumed to be $4,865,000 for 1995 and 1996.
XYZ's Maximum Annual Debt Service is assumed to be $5,617,000 for 1995 and 1996.

facility's total excess margin will exceed its operating margin by 2–5 percent.

The operating ratio measures a facility's ability to adequately cover its cash operating expenses with its cash operating revenues. The removal of noncash expenses (i.e., depreciation and amortization) from the numerator is offset by the removal of noncash revenues (i.e., earned entrance fees) from the denominator. This ratio provides a better gauge of a facility's operating profitability than the operating margin ratio. A mature facility that is operating efficiently should have an operating ratio of less than 100 percent.

Capital structure and cash flow ratios

Capital structure ratios determine balance sheet strengths and weaknesses by relating various capital structure components to each other. Cash flow ratios provide an indication of a facility's ability to cover its annual debt-service requirements with its net available cash.

The unrestricted cash and investments to long-term debt ratio measures a facility's unrestricted cash as a percentage of long-term debt. Unrestricted cash includes board-designated funds, trustee-held funds only when earmarked for operating reserves, and donations set aside for operations. CCRCs need to develop cash balances so they can cover unplanned expenses, cover health care liabilities, and fund future expansion and renovation. An unrestricted cash and investments to long-term debt ratio greater than 30 percent is favorable.

Debt-service coverage ratios are widely viewed by analysts as one of the most important gauges of a facility's strength. The debt-service coverage ratio-unadjusted measures a CCRC's ability to cover its annual debt-service with net available cash. In order to arrive at the numerator for this ratio, noncash revenues are subtracted from and noncash expenses are added to change in unrestricted net assets; interest expense is also added since it is included in the denominator. Net entrance fees collected are added as well. As a conservative measure, analysts prefer to use maximum annual debt-service in the denominator rather than actual annual debt-service. It is common for a mature, well-run facility to achieve a debt-service coverage ratio-unadjusted of greater than 1.5x.

The debt-service coverage ratio-adjusted indicates a facility's reliance on entrance fees to cover its annual debt-service. By removing net entrance fees collected from the numerator, the impact of apartment turnover and apartment fill-up on cash flow is neutralized. A mature facility that relies on revenue from entrance fees to pay debt-service (rental facilities do not rely on entrance fees) might exceed a debt-service coverage ratio-adjusted of .75x.

By comparing long-term debt to long-term debt plus unrestricted fund balance, the debt to capitalization ratio measures a facility's reliance on debt versus retained earnings and contributed capital. It is acceptable for a facility, especially a startup, to have a debt to capitalization ratio in excess of 100 percent, or it may even be negative. Such ratios are possible if a new facility has not been operating long enough to amortize deferred revenue from entrance fees to its statement of activities.

Debt-service as a percentage of total revenue and nonoperating gains indicates the portion of total revenues and gains allocated to payment of annual debt-service. A high debt-service as a percentage of total revenue and nonoperating gains ratio can signify a facility's excessive debt burden. It is acceptable for a young facility that relied on debt to finance its original construction to have a debt-service as a percentage of total revenue and nonoperating gains ratio greater than 20 percent. A well-run, mature facility, however, will have a debt-service as a percentage of total revenue and nonoperating gains ratio of less than 15 percent.

Liquidity ratios

Liquidity ratios gauge a facility's ability to meet unforeseen needs for cash. The definition of unrestricted cash is the same for liquidity ratios as it is for unrestricted cash and investments to long-term debt. Two ratios used to measure a facility's cash position are the days cash on hand ratio and the cushion ratio.

The days cash on hand ratio measures the number of days a facility can cover its operating expenses given its unrestricted cash balance. In other words, if a facility with a days cash on hand ratio of 120 experiences an operating crisis, and has lost its source of revenues, it will be able to cover its operating expenses for 120 days from its cash reserves. A well-run facility will have an unrestricted cash balance of at least 100 days.

The cushion ratio has recently gained favor by credit analysts as a measure of cash position. It indicates the number of times a facility's unrestricted cash can cover its maximum annual debt-service. For instance, a cushion ratio of 4.8x implies that a facility's unrestricted cash can cover its maximum annual debt-service 4.8 times.

CASE STUDY: XYZ

To illustrate the fundamental issues related to analyzing a CCRC credit, a case study of a hypothetical CCRC, XYZ,[8] has been created. To facilitate this analysis, XYZ's ratios have been calculated and compared to the Fitch and CCAC medians. It is important to recognize that while this analysis focuses on the financial strengths and weakness of XYZ, other factors such as management and board experience, facility location, and competitive pressures are equally important in evaluating its overall strength. Table 2 provides a summary of XYZ's financial statements.

Background of XYZ

XYZ is a nonprofit CCRC established in 1990. It consists of 400 independent living units (ILUs), 20 assisted living units (ALUs), and 60 skilled nursing beds. XYZ has benefited from minimal competition and an average occu-

pancy exceeding 95 percent during the last three years. The facility's management is experienced and competent. Its change in unrestricted assets has shown steady, marked improvement. Its board of directors has been effective in directing the facility's goals.

XYZ, looking to reduce its interest expense, now wishes to refund its outstanding $59,500,000 of Series 1990 unrated tax-exempt bonds, originally issued for the construction of the facility.

Three factors influencing the economic feasibility of XYZ's refunding are (1) the current interest rate environment compared to the interest rate environment in 1990, (2) the optional redemption provisions of the Series 1990 bonds, and (3) the ability of XYZ to obtain a stand-alone rating. Obviously, lower interest rates, flexible redemption provisions, and a conversion of the Series 1997 bonds from unrated to rated all increase the likelihood of an economically feasible refunding. For this analysis, the impact of interest rates and the Series 1990 bond's optional redemption provisions are not considered; the focus of this analysis will be on XYZ's ability to obtain a rating.

Analysis of XYZ

In order for a credit analysis to be meaningful, it is necessary to review at least two years of a facility's operating history. Two years of predictable performance form the basis of a trend. If there is significant disparity between years, further analysis may be required. If, however, ratios are consistent between the years, it is acceptable to focus on just the most recent year. XYZ's ratios are consistent; therefore, unless noted, our analysis centers on its most recent fiscal year, 1996. XYZ's financial ratios are summarized and compared to the Fitch and CCAC medians in Table 1.

Table 2. XYZ's Financial Statements

Statement Of Changes In Unrestricted Net Assets (Income Statement) (000's)			Statement of financial position (balance sheet) (000's)		
	1995	1996		1995	1996
Operating revenues			Assets		
Service revenue	$ 9,780	$10,496	Cash and investments-unrestricted	$24,551	$25,164
Earned entrance fees	3,050	3,232			
Investment income	2,515	2,814	Cash and investments-restricted	14,689	15,838
Total operating revenues	**15,345**	**16,542**	Accounts receivable	2,347	2,291
			Property, plant & equipment, net	50,961	50,665
Operating expenses			Debt issuance costs, net	1,648	1,558
Operations	8,180	8,922	Other assets	1,609	1,251
Depreciation and amortization	2,182	2,269	**Total Assets**	**$95,805**	**$96,767**
Interest	4,942	4,884			
Total operating expenses	**15,304**	**16,075**	Liabilities		
			Current liabilities	$1,974	$2,120
Operating income	41	467	Deferred revenue	24,903	25,615
			Refundable entrance fees	21,009	20,868
Nonoperating revenues			Long-term debt	59,950	59,500
Unrealized gains	859	480	Other	1,698	1,340
Gain on sale of assets	250	150	Total liabilities	109,534	109,443
Nonoperating income	1,109	630	Unrestricted net assets	(13,729)	(12,676)
Change in unrestricted net assets	**1,150**	**1,097**	**Total liabilities and net assets**	**$95,805**	**$96,767**

Profitability

XYZ demonstrates considerable operating strengths. Its operating margin ratio of 2.8 percent and total excess margin of 6.4 percent exceed the CCAC and Fitch medians.

XYZ's operating strength can be attributed to a number of factors. First, it has maintained an adequate pricing structure, increasing the cost of its ILUs and ALUs 4–7 percent annually. Its skilled nursing fees have also been adjusted annually to outpace rising nursing expenses.

Second, its nursing payer mix has remained very favorable: 50 percent private pay, 15 percent Medicare, 35 percent Medicaid. (A higher percentage of private pay is desirable. The nursing industry average is 34 percent private pay, 58 percent Medicaid, and 8 percent Medicare and other.)[9]

Third, XYZ's investments have benefited from the bull market of 1996. Its investment income, included in operating revenue, increased nearly 12 percent from 1995 to 1996. As a result of these three factors, operating revenue rose 8 percent from 1995 to 1996. Operating expenses rose 5 percent.

XYZ's operating ratio at 103.7 percent is weaker than the Fitch (100.0%) and CCAC (102.7%) medians. A ratio greater than 100 percent can indicate a facility's undesirable reliance on entrance fees to cover operating expenses. XYZ's operating ratio for 1996 improved 3 percent over 1995. If this trend continues in 1997, its operating ratio will be as strong as the Fitch and CCAC medians.

Capital structure

XYZ's capital structure ratios present the weakest side of its financial picture. Its debt-service coverage ratio of 1.65 falls below both the Fitch (2.32) and CCAC (2.00) medians. And its debt-service coverage ratio-adjusted of .78 falls between the Fitch (.73) and CCAC (1.10) medians.

Its debt-service coverage ratio, which had been above 1.80 in prior years, has dropped. Low apartment turnover during 1995 and 1996, partially mitigated by an increase in unrestricted net assets, reduced the amount of cash XYZ received from entrance fees. XYZ's apartment turnover should be monitored.

XYZ's cash to debt ratios showed improvement from 1995 (41%) to 1996 (42%). The Series 1997 refunding will slightly increase annual principal payments, but this increase should be offset as XYZ builds its cash balances.

Compared to the Fitch (64%) and CCAC (74%) medians, XYZ's debt to capital ratio of 127 percent is high. Its negative fund balance is responsible for its high debt to capital ratio. A negative trend in fund balance can be a sign that a facility is losing money. While XYZ has a negative fund balance—it incurred some planned losses for the first three years of operations (until occupancy was stabilized), and then booked some extraordinary losses—its fund balance has been improving. Furthermore, as mentioned before, a new facility such as XYZ, in its fourth year of operation, has not had enough time to fully amortize its deferred revenue to its statement of activities.

XYZ's debt-service as a percentage of total revenue and nonoperating gains ratio of 33 percent is its weakest ratio. Fitch's median is 11 percent and CCAC's median is 9 percent. The reason for its high debt-service as a percentage of total revenue and nonoperating gains is XYZ's $59,500,000 of outstanding Series 1990 bonds. The Series 1997 refunding combined with strong operating performance will improve this ratio. This ratio should be reevaluated when and if XYZ explores raising additional capital for improvements or expansion.

Cash position

XYZ's unrestricted cash has grown steadily since the facility began operations, averaging 2–10 percent annually. Unrestricted cash increased 3 percent from 1995 to 1996. In addition to healthy profit margins, because of the efforts of its fund-raising staff and volunteers, XYZ has been the beneficiary of significant restricted and unrestricted contributions.

These factors have placed XYZ in a strong cash position. Its days cash on hand ratio of 665 is exceptional. It well exceeds the Fitch (241) and CCAC (182) medians. In fact, it exceeds Fitch's highest rating category ("A") by more than 300 days.[6]

While XYZ's cushion ratio of 4.5 is below Fitch's median of 5.x,[10] its cushion ratio is not a concern. Taking into consideration that XYZ is refunding its Series 1990 bonds—with the intent of obtaining lower interest rates, and in turn, lowering its annual debt-service payments—its cushion ratio will improve in 1997.

Results of XYZ credit analysis

When comparing XYZ to the Fitch and CCAC medians, we recognize its many strengths and few weaknesses. Its operations exhibit a positive trend that will continue to add to its already healthy cash balances. And while XYZ's capital structure ratios depict a young facility faced with the challenges of retiring debt and minimizing the impact of start-up losses and unamortized entrance fees, there is little cause for further inspection; its continued operating strength, strict monitoring of its apartment turnover, and proposed refinancing will do much to ameliorate these weaknesses. Facility XYZ will likely receive an investment grade rating.

FUTURE TRENDS IN CCRC CREDIT ANALYSIS

During the past four years, the Financial Accounting Standards Board (FASB) has issued three Statements that will affect CCRCs' financial ratios: FASB 116, FASB 117, and FASB 124. Because many CCRCs have avoided converting their financial statement format until required, we are in 1998 just beginning to see the impact of these FASB Statements.

FASB 116 and 117

FASB 116 and 117, *Accounting for Contributions Received and Contributions Made* and *Financial Statements of Not-for-Profit Organizations,* establish standards for contributions and financial statement format, respectively. Historically, there has been little differentiation between contribution types; contributions were not required to be classified based on their degree of restriction. With FASB 116 and 117, contributions, as well as other revenues, expenses, gains, and losses, must be categorized as unrestricted, temporarily unrestricted, or permanently restricted.[11,12]

While FASB 117 allows additional classifications under these three categories (i.e., operating and nonoperating), the accounting profession has predominantly adopted the format outlined in paragraph 59 of FASB 117.[12] This format divides the statement of activities into two main sections: (1) total unrestricted revenues and gains and (2) total expenses and losses. The adopted format does not make a distinction between operating and nonoperating revenues and expenses.

Because the adopted format does not distinguish between operating and nonoperating revenues and expenses, profitability ratios that rely on such a distinction become blurred. For instance, the inclusion of contributions in total unrestricted revenues and gains (formerly, operating revenue) improves a CCRC's operating ratio and operating margin. It also blurs the distinction between operating margin and total excess margin.

To develop a meaningful distinction between operating and nonoperating ratios, a credit analyst will have to separate operating and nonoperating items (as has been done in XYZ's case study) or, alternatively, the credit community will rely on new ratios. For instance, it is possible that the operating margin and total excess margin ratios will be combined into a new ratio (i.e., change in unrestricted net assets divided by total unrestricted revenues and gains).

FASB 124

FASB 124, *Accounting for Certain Investments Held by Not-for-Profit Organizations,* requires investments to be reported at fair market value (formerly, investments were reported as lesser of cost or market).[13] Under FASB 124, any appreciation of a facility's investment portfolio from a previous year's will be recorded on the statement of activities as an unrealized gain or loss.

This accounting change will have no impact on capital structure ratios such as the debt-service coverage ratios, because the unrealized gain or loss as a noncash item would be excluded from those ratios. The liquidity ratios also would not be impacted. However, the profitability ratios would be. During market upswings or downswings, a CCRC's total excess margin would be reflective of market conditions, and not necessarily operating performance. Again, the credit community is currently deliberating over how to treat this item. One suggestion has been to exclude unrealized investment gains and losses from this ratio.

• • •

As the nonprofit CCRC industry grows, it will receive more attention from the credit community. Credit analysts, taking advantage of the latest analytical tools, will be able to quickly unravel a CCRC's financial statements and paint an accurate picture of its strengths and weaknesses. As a result, the nonprofit CCRC community will see a continuation of a trend that started in 1989: nonprofit CCRCs will demonstrate stronger credit profiles, obtain more ratings, and improve their access to capital markets.

NOTES

1. *Securities Data and Ziegler Securities' Senior Living Group Database,* June 1997 (http://www.bcziegler.com).

2. Population Division, U.S. Bureau of the Census. *Population Estimates Program.* Suitland, MD: Author, 1996.

3. The number of ratings issued by Fitch Investors Services, Standard and Poor's Corporation, and Moody's is as of June 1997.

4. Annett, J.M., et al. *Financial Ratios & Trend Analysis of CCAC Accredited Communities.* Washington, DC: American Association of Homes and Services for the Aging, 1996.

5. The CCAC study includes 91 single-site and 26 multisite facilities.

6. Merrigan, E.C. *Health Care Financial Ratio Medians.* New York, NY: Fitch Investors Service, 1996.

7. Merrigan, E.C. *Rating Guidelines for Nonprofit Continuing Care Retirement Communities.* New York, NY: Fitch Investors Service, 1994.

8. XYZ facility was created for purposes of this case study only; any resemblance to other CCRCs is coincidental.

9. SMG Marketing Group, 1993.

10. The CCAC did not include the cushion ratio in its 1996 publication. This ratio will be included in its 1997 publication.

11. Financial Accounting Standards Board. *Statement No. 116: Accounting for Contributions Received and Contributions Made.* Norwalk, CT: FASB, June 1993.

12. Financial Accounting Standards Board. *Statement No. 117: Financial Statements of Not-for-Profit Organizations.* Norwalk, CT: FASB, June 1993.

13. Financial Accounting Standards Board. *Statement No. 124: Accounting for Certain Investments Held by Not-for-Profit Organizations.* Norwalk, CT: FASB, November 1995.

CHAPTER 17

Mini-Case Study 2: Changing Economic Realities in the Health Care Setting: A Physician's Office Teaching Case That Includes Specifics on Changing Payment Levels

Improving Patient Care in a Changing Environment: A Teaching Case*

William B. Weeks, MD, MBA

CASE PRESENTATION

Bob Collins looked across his desk with an air of frustration. It was 9:15 PM; he had been in the office all day, had seen 47 patients, and had answered innumerable phone calls. His desk was piled high with the incomplete charts from the day's patients, and he still had about half of them left to complete. Bob knew that the challenge of the next several hours would be in keeping his patients straight. With some dismay, Bob wondered if he was providing the best quality care, as he tried to remember patient presentations, lab tests ordered, and treatment plans developed from hours ago.

This chaos was not what Bob had anticipated when he completed his fellowship in geriatrics 4 years ago. He thought that he would be able to dedicate a large proportion of his time to geriatric patient care, having an adequate amount of time in each encounter to assess fully the complexity of his patient's needs, and that he would be well paid for this specialized knowledge. He thought he had found such an idealized practice in a semirural setting.

For the first year, Bob's practice was what he had anticipated. The large majority of his patients were older adults; he averaged 15 patient visits per workday; he could charge a premium for his specialized knowledge; and he had Thursdays off. Bob was the only geriatrician in his area, which supported a population base of 22,000. Managed care had not infiltrated the area and represented only 12% of the market. Bob had no managed care patients, and 95% of his income was derived from fee-for-service indemnity plans. He had a 6-month waiting list for patients who wished to have him as their geriatrician—patients who would gladly wait the 6 months to access his specialized knowledge. He received consultation requests from both of the large group practices in his area—Group West and Group East—neither of which was staffed with a geriatrician. He had admitting privileges at the local not-for-profit hospital, a small community-based hospital with 60 beds and an in-house, multilevel nursing home. He did consulting work for the nursing home about 1 day per week.

However, because of an increasingly competitive market, things had dramatically changed over the last 4 years. After his first year in practice, a regional health maintenance organization (HMO) began to compete

*Source: Reprinted from W.B. Weeks, Improving Patient Care in a Changing Environment: A Teaching Case, *Journal of Ambulatory Care Management,* Vol. 21, No. 3, pp. 49–55, © 1998, Aspen Publishers, Inc.

aggressively for patients in the area. The HMO had an affiliation with an academic center 45 miles away, which housed a geriatric residency program and was staffed with numerous subspecialists, including three geriatricians, two geriatric psychiatrists, and a geriatric nutritionist. The local practitioners were clearly encouraged to refer to the affiliate by the HMO, but there still seemed to be enough geriatric patients who wished to receive local care. Bob's waiting list had dropped to 2 months, but things were still good.

However, the market for HMOs had become increasingly more competitive. There were now four regional and national HMOs in the market, dividing 62% of the patient population. This came as a result of three major employers in the area encouraging employees and retirees to sign up with a lower cost HMO plan. The two group practices in the area competed heavily for the HMO volume, now accounting for one third of the population. The salaries of the practitioners in both group practices suffered as a result of withholdings and capitation.

The impact on Bob's practice was great (Table 1). He initially resisted joining forces with either of the group practices, as they each contributed to about one half of his patient load through referrals. However, within 6 months, Bob felt as though he had no choice. He had seen his geriatrics practice dwindle to the point where he needed the additional income from general internal medicine patients to support his life style. He joined Group West as a half-time generalist, with the hope that he could specialize within the group as a geriatrician. He discovered that the volume per day required for profitability was so high that the complex geriatrics cases he initially took on considerably affected his productivity. In his first complete year with the group, he did not get any of the holdback/ bonus for his HMO work. As a result, over the next 6 months, he attempted to trim his geriatric caseload by agreeing to see an increasing proportion of general internal medicine patients.

In addition, there had been a major impact on Bob's geriatric private practice and his relationship with the hospital. Upon his joining Group West, his referrals from Group East stopped. Group East had to make better use of the academic resources available through its affiliate for referrals. It was clear that the camaraderie that had existed between the

Table 1 A Summary of Changes in Bob's Practice over the Past 5 Years

Bob's Practice	1992	1997
% geriatric patients	75	35
Number of scheduled visits per day	15	28
Overbooks	3	10
Waiting list	6 mos	3 weeks
No-show rate	8%	20%
AM	8%	35%
PM	8%	7%
Bob's net income	$143,000	$145,000
% of Bob's net income from indemnity plans	95%	30%
% of Bob's income from managed care	0%	65%
% income from Hospital Care Services	25%	6%

groups had vanished in the competitive atmosphere. Bob was also concerned that an additional geriatrician in the area would only increase the impact on his practice, as Group East might become more aggressive in pursuing the geriatric population. While Bob had previously spent 1 day a week consulting to the hospital-based nursing home, he now managed only a few cases sporadically, generally patients who were not well covered by insurance or were poorly reimbursed through a state payment mechanism. The local not-for-profit hospital had developed an affiliation with the academic medical center, decreasing its bed capacity to 35 beds and eliminating one half of the nursing home. Selected demographic and economic changes in the region are shown in Table 2.

The complexities rose exponentially when Bob considered the actual seeing of patients. From a patient care perspective, Bob was concerned about the results of a recent survey that examined patient satisfaction with care (Figure 1). Of particular concern were the complaints of excessive waiting times experienced by Bob's patients. Before all the changes, Bob thought that a busy waiting room was the sign of a productive, caring provider. Now Bob was confronted with the reality that patients were leaving his practice because of having to spend hours in his waiting room. He knew that he could become more efficient with the processing of patients,

but it seemed that he often encountered the famous "doorknob questions." These complex, time-consuming questions were usually the primary motivations for the patient visit and were expressed by the patient just as Bob was leaving the room. Another problem was his no-show rate. On any given day, 25% of his patients would not show up or would be considerably late, usually because they forgot the appointment. This created a backlog because Bob had to "work the patient in" and catch up with patients who needed to be seen.

Bob's work life was challenging from a staffing perspective as well. Because Bob's private practice office was located in the same complex as Group West, he saw both his private patients and the Group West patients in his own office space. While the original agreement had called for a 50/50 split in office expenses, Bob's private practice was diminishing. He was spending more time in the Group West practice to maintain productivity standards, making a 75/25 split appear more realistic. He supported one nurse practitioner from his private practice income, and he was provided one nurse practitioner from Group West, who was only appointed on a rotating basis. Therefore, for most of the patients seen by the Group West nurse practitioner, Bob had to carefully review the encounters and be more available than he felt he should have to be. Most of this careful review came at the end of the day, after the nurse

Table 2 A Summary of Selected Changes in Regional Demographics over the Past 5 Years

Regional Demographics	1992	1997
Population of catchment area	22,000	25,000
Percentage of population over 65	14%	14%
Median income	$35,000	$37,000
Physicians per 100,000	205	167
Beds per 1,000	2	1.4
HMO penetration	12%	62%

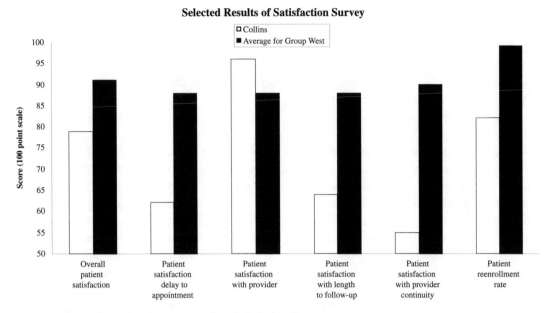

Figure 1 Selected Results of a Recent Patient Satisfaction Survey

practitioner had left, leaving Bob to correct oversights on his own. There were problems with chart content and chart access, and Bob did not have data readily available about the plan to which a particular patient might belong. This became particularly complex since a number of the HMOs had launched Medicare managed care products, and the patients could change plans month to month but keep the same provider. Although Bob considered it unethical to treat patients differently based on their health care plan, it was evident that there were financial incentives that did not differentiate patient care but that did affect his and the patient's income, such as which generic antibiotic was reimbursable to the patient in each plan or which plans would reimburse for which chemistry profiles. The result was that Bob tried to review the charts at the end of every day to rectify problems, taking an inordinate amount of time and generally resulting in few gains. He knew that his man-

agement of patient flow was not optimal but wondered how to improve it.

Bob was frustrated. His efforts to work harder only resulted in his spending more time at the office. He knew the system needed to be reworked, but he did not have the capital to automate all the charts. He also knew that the population, given the referral streams to the academic center, could not tolerate an additional geriatrician without adversely affecting his patient stream further. After a quick call to his home to wish the kids goodnight, he returned to his charts, disgruntled, wondering why he had chosen the practice of medicine in the first place. What could he do to make things better?

CASE ANALYSIS

This complex case examines the impact of changing economic realities in the health care setting. Bob Collins' case is not unique to providers. Some of the problems in his practice seem obvious and easily solved; however, Bob is hesitant to invest even more time in the running of his practice, despite a realization that such an initial investment would pay off. The author will examine the case from three perspectives and make recommendations.

It is useful to consider the case from an "inside-out" vantage point. Figure 2 describes a conceptual model of health care. The patient and clinician perspectives are represented as "inside" the system, and external factors, such as government, business, and insurers, are depicted as "outside" the system. Bob's practice transformation has largely been a result of his response to external pressures: the changing health care marketplace and changes in the local medical economy. Bob may have little direct impact on "outside in" forces, but he has failed to respond to these forces in a productive manner. His focus has been from the provider and insurer perspective, almost to the exclusion of the patient or consumer perspective. Looking at the case from three perspectives and making recommendations for improvement will show how the "inside out" paradigm works from a consumer's point of view.

CUSTOMER PERSPECTIVE

Patients who are generally healthy and value their time probably would not want to be a patient in Bob's practice. A provider who cares for a panel of patients under any type of risk system (whether capitation or bonus incentive) needs a mix of healthy and sick patients to have a successful practice. The inefficiencies inherent in Bob's practice are likely to create an adverse selection problem: the patients who are more ill, who are more reliant on the physician, and who may value time less will probably be satisfied with Bob—after all, he is a considerate, highly skilled physician. However, those who are less ill, are less reliant on the health care system, and value time outside the waiting room will probably seek another provider.

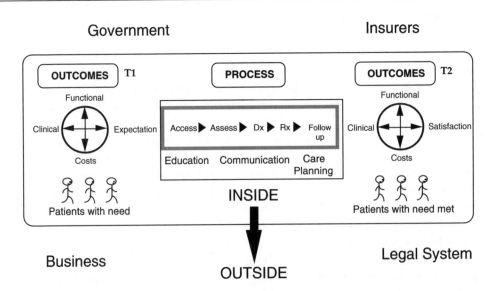

Figure 2 A Conceptual Model of Health Care with the Perspective of What Lies "Inside" and "Outside" the System of Care

Bob's inefficient practice style, with little apparent regard for patient time, will hamper him further, because only the most ill will continue in his practice.

The lack of consistency among nurse practitioners would be an additional concern for patients. It would be beneficial for the patient to develop a relationship with a single midlevel provider. This relationship would improve Bob's practice efficiency as well, because there would be less wasted time, as nurse practitioners would not have to review the case and history at each visit. The patient would value a personal touch—the recognition of the nurse practitioner who knew the patient and his or her case.

Finally, Bob could win patients if he were to add additional value to their visit. As is stated in the case, the Medicare HMO policies would allow patients to keep Bob as a provider, regardless of their plan choice. For instance, if Bob were to provide educational health maintenance videos in his office, he could provide valuable information, giving patients less of a sense of wasted time. Further, the "doorknob" questions might be reduced, as the patient could gain information on "doorknob" topics without using as much of Bob's time. For the relatively small cost of a video player, television, and informational tapes, Bob could increase his patients' knowledge and improve their care.

ORGANIZATIONAL PERSPECTIVE

From Group West's perspective, Bob is a cost center. However, he may more than compensate for his own lack of profitability by providing valuable family services in a one-stop fashion. The value to Group West is Bob's geriatric expertise, his strong personality, and his ability to round out Group West's capacity to treat all ages. If Group West is like most other practices, it recognizes that engagement of the entire family leads to a more efficient practice and customer loyalty. These efficiencies are enhanced through the convenience offered to customers who do all of their medical marketing at one center, making the building space that Group West rents to a local pharmacy more valuable.

However, because of Bob's inefficient practice style and the changing mix of patients to a younger age group, Group West is losing most of Bob's value. Group West also faces a challenge from Group East, which is promoting its affiliated geriatrics expertise and may be recruiting their own geriatrician. Group West needs to improve Bob's customer orientation to maintain the market share and reputation it has.

First, Group West should provide a reliable nurse practitioner for Bob, making his practice more efficient. Second, Group West should offer to buy Bob's entire practice. Part of his practice difficulties are due to his management of the private part of his practice. This internal management is inefficient, and scale economies could be achieved through a single management of practices. Finally, after Bob's practice is integrated, Group West should leverage Bob's skill as a geriatrician more effectively. By targeting the entire family and promoting Bob's geriatric expertise, Group West could expect less "production" by Bob, improve customer value and loyalty, and maintain a family and community relationship and, therefore, increase profitability.

PROVIDER PERSPECTIVE

Bob appears to be miserable. He is frustrated by the rework he has to do as an inherent part of his practice. Until his practice system changes, Bob will continue in the same path, gradually losing his competitive advantage.

Bob needs to examine his practice from a customer perspective, both Group West's and his own. He needs to invest effort in improving patient care at a process level. He spends so much of his time doing rework that a minimal investment in process reengineering would have a terrific payoff.

Many of the suggestions from the previous sections would be important for him to consider. Of great concern is Bob's almost exclusive focus on his own bottom line. Customers pay for quality, even in health care. Within Bob's practice, the most ill clearly value him and pay with their time. However, Bob is not leveraging the assets he brings to the practice. He should change his perspective from a focus on a stable income to a focus on enhancing value to the customer. With this focus, a stable income can take care of itself.

●   ●   ●

The author has presented a case and has examined the case from three different perspectives. It is important to note that customer value is a goal common to all three perspectives: the customer wants value; the organization needs to enhance customer value to remain profitable; and, if Bob enhances customer value of the patients he treats, he can keep those patients. The case demonstrates the complexities of providing medical care in a changing environment. However, the case also demonstrates that much of the ability to enhance customer value rests with the practitioners and the internal systems managers. Managed care is not necessarily an evil force; many of the "evils" are poorly planned responses to a changing environment. The good news is that through a customer orientation, system redesign, and value enhancement, managed care can be managed.

RBRVS—1999 Update*

Jon Harris-Shapiro and Marcia S. Greenstein

Medicare RBRVS has become widely used as a standard for physician fee scales by both traditional health insurance plans and managed care organizations. There are significant variations in the way RBRVS has been adapted by these private payers. These variations, when combined with annual changes Medicare has made to the underlying components of RBRVS, may result in unintended and unexpected increases in physician payments. To avoid surprises, payers using RBRVS-based fee scales need to carefully evaluate the overall impact of annual RBRVS modifications on their delivery systems. Key words: *health plan, managed care, Medicare RBRVS, physician fee scales, physician reimbursement, provider payments*

Since Medicare implemented its Resource Based Relative Value Scale (RBRVS), an increasing number of health plans and managed care organizations have changed to physician fee scales that are based on RBRVS. As a result, the marketplace has virtually made Medicare RBRVS a national standard for physician fees. Medicare makes significant changes to the RBRVS system and its associated payment levels each year. *Private payers with RBRVS-based fee scales need to carefully evaluate the impact of these annual changes on their own expenditures, especially when their fee scales use some of the RBRVS components and not others.*

Medicare's RBRVS formula for 1999 consists of the following components: Conversion Factors (CFs), Relative Value Units (RVUs), and Geographic Cost Practice Indices (GPCIs). For each service code, fees are computed using the following formula:

$$CF \times [(RVU_{work} \times GPCI_{work}) + (RVU_{practice\ expense} \times GPCI_{practice\ expense}) + RVU_{malpractice} \times GPCI_{malpractice})]$$

A number of methodologies have been established for using RBRVS as the basis for private payer fee scales. These methodologies differ in the application of the components of RBRVS. Typical variations include separate market-based conversion factors by specialty group and exclusion of the geographic cost practice indices. Medicare's changes to the RBRVS components are interdependent; adopting them piecemeal can produce unintended, adverse consequences.

LESSONS FROM PRIOR YEARS

Medicare introduced the Work Adjuster in 1997 as a temporary factor to achieve budget neutrality. Payers that did not include this adjustment in their fee updates saw physician

Source: Reprinted from J. Harris-Shapiro and Marcia S. Greenstein, RBRVS—1999 Update, *Journal of Health Care Finance,* Vol. 26, No. 2 (in press) © 1999, Aspen Publishers, Inc.

expenditures increase by 5% to 8%.

In 1998, Medicare introduced a site-of-service differential. For private payers, the impact of this differential depended on their mix between facility and office-based services. Some health plans reported that the 1998 RVU changes increased their physician payments by 2% to 4%. This increase would have translated to approximately $110,000 per year for a health plan with 10,000 non-Medicare covered lives.

CHANGES FOR 1999

The basic formula for computing 1999 fees is shown above. There are a number of modifications from 1998 that need to be evaluated:

- *Conversion Factor:* The 1999 physician fee schedule conversion factor *decreased* 5.3% from $36.6873 to $34.7315. This decrease reflects the net effect of two adjustments. The first adjustment *increased* the conversion factor by 2.3% to reflect the change in the Medicare Economic Index. The second adjustment *decreased* the factor by 7.46% due to the combined effect of several items, including the elimination of the Work Adjuster. It is important to note that the reduction in the conversion factor is necessary to offset increases in Medicare payments that would have otherwise resulted from changes made to other components of the RBRVS formula. *Private payers may need to make similar adjustments to their conversion factors to avoid an unintended increase in expenditures.*
- *Work Adjuster:* As discussed above, the explicit Work Adjuster factor of .917 has been removed from the fee computation formula. Instead it has been incorporated

into the revised RVUs and the conversion factor.

- *Practice Expense RVU:* 1999 marks the beginning of a four-year transition from charge-based practice expense RVUs to resource-based practice expense RVUs, as shown in Table 1. The site-of-service differential introduced in 1998 is still applicable for many services that may be performed in both facility and non-facility settings. The differential lowers fees for facility-based services to exclude physician practice costs.
- *GPCIs:* The impact of using updated GPCIs ranges from −1.1 to +1.2% compared to 1998.
- *Anesthesia:* The anesthesia conversion factor is defined as 46% of the physician fee schedule conversion factor. This calculation yields $17.24 for 1999.

IMPLEMENTATION ISSUES

The anticipated impact of implementing the 1999 fee update should be carefully evaluated, including the effect on costs, network configuration, and provider agreements:

- *Overall Cost:* The 1999 changes to the Medicare Physician Fee Schedule will increase payments about 2% to 3%. This reflects the combined impact of a decrease in the conversion factor and an

Table 1 Transition from Charge-Based RVUs to Resource-Based RVUs by Year

Year	Charge-Based RVUs	Resource-Based RVUs
1999	75%	25%
2000	50%	50%
2001	25%	75%
2002+	0%	100%

overall increase in the RVUs. Health plans that adopt the 1999 RVUs and do not reduce their conversion factor will see costs increase about 8.5%. For private payers, market-based conversion factors, non-Medicare distribution of services, and other operational issues may produce different results. Given budget pressures in most health plans and managed care organizations, it is important that private payers carefully determine the overall impact of the 1999 RVU changes on their fee scale.

- *Resource Based Physician Expense RVUs:* Table 2, adapted from the *Federal Register,* shows the impact on Medicare payments by specialty of the transition to resource-based RVUs. This comparison excludes the effects of the annual updates to the conversion factor. As shown in column one, the annual impact of the transition on Medicare payments ranges from –4% for gastroenterology to +6% for optometry. The cumulative 4-year impact, reflecting the full transition to resource-based physician expense RVUs, is shown in the second column. In general, those specialties that furnish more office-based services are expected to experience larger increases in payments than those specialties that furnish less office-based services.
- *Cost by Procedure:* Table 3 shows the percentage change in both RVU factors and Medicare fees from 1998 to 1999 for several high-volume procedures for facility and non-facility sites of service.
- *Network Configuration:* The magnitude of the impact of the transition to resource-based RVUs will depend on both the mix of services provided and where those services are performed. Private payers will need to determine whether the site-of-service payment differential

Table 2 Resource-Based Practice Expense Relative Value Units Change in Medicare Payments by Selected Specialties

Specialty	Impact per Year	Cumulative 4-Year Impact
Optometry	6%	27%
Dermatology	5%	20%
Rheumatology	4%	16%
Otolaryngology	2%	9%
Podiatry	2%	9%
Family Practice	2%	7%
Hematology/ Oncology	2%	6%
Urology	1%	5%
General Practice	1%	4%
Obstetrics/ Gynecology	1%	4%
Ophthalmology	1%	4%
Internal Medicine	0%	2%
Other Physician	0%	1%
Psychiatry	0%	1%
Anesthesiology	0%	0%
Neurology	0%	–1%
Pulmonary	–1%	–4%
Radiation Oncology	–2%	–6%
General Surgery	–2%	–7%
Nephrology	–2%	–7%
Chiropractic	–2%	–8%
Cardiology	–2%	–9%
Emergency Medicine	–3%	–10%
Radiology	–3%	–10%
Neurosurgery	–3%	–11%
Vascular Surgery	–3%	–11%
Cardiac Surgery	–3%	–12%
Thoracic Surgery	–3%	–12%
Pathology	–3%	–13%
Gastroenterology	–4%	–15%

Note: Excludes effect of annual updates to conversion factor.
Source: Reprinted from 63 *Federal Register,* 58,894–58,895.

will impact physician behavior. Physicians may tend to perform certain services in the office that had previously been done in a facility setting because of the higher non-facility payment. Networks with a disproportionately high volume of office services could see pay-

Table 3 Comparison of 1998 and1999 RVUs and Medicare Fees High-Volume Codes

CPT Code	Description	% Change from 1998 to 1999					
		Non-Facility Site of Service			Facility Site of Service		
		RVUs	Conv Factor	Fees	RVUs	Conv Factor	Fees
56308	Laproscopy; hysterectomy	na	na	na	2.3%	−5.3%	−3.2%
59400	Obstetric care	4.1%	−5.3%	−1.4%	4.1%	−5.3%	−1.4%
59510	Caesarean delivery	na	na	na	4.3%	−5.3%	−1.3%
69436	Create eardrum opening	3.2%	−5.3%	−2.3%	3.2%	−5.3%	−2.3%
70553	Magnetic image, brain	6.5%	−5.3%	0.8%	6.5%	−5.3%	0.8%
71020	Chest X-ray	5.9%	−5.3%	0.3%	5.9%	−5.3%	0.3%
72148	Magnetic image, lumbar spine	6.4%	−5.3%	0.7%	6.4%	−5.3%	0.7%
76805	Echo exam of pregnant uterus	5.5%	−5.3%	−0.2%	5.5%	−5.3%	−0.2%
92004	Eye exam, new patient	20.6%	−5.3%	14.1%	13.9%	−5.3%	7.9%
99202	Office/outpatient visit, new	14.9%	−5.3%	8.7%	14.8%	−5.3%	8.7%
99203	Office/outpatient visit, est	16.3%	−5.3%	10.1%	15.3%	−5.3%	9.1%
99212	Office/outpatient visit, est	14.9%	−5.3%	8.8%	14.8%	−5.3%	8.7%
99213	Office/outpatient visit, est	11.7%	−5.3%	5.7%	12.4%	−5.3%	6.4%
99214	Office/outpatient visit, est	13.2%	−5.3%	7.2%	13.6%	−5.3%	7.5%
99223	Initial hospital care	na	na	na	8.4%	−5.3%	2.7%
	All Services	11.0%	−5.3%	5.0%	5.0%	−5.3%	−0.5%
	Both Sites of Service				8.5%	−5.3%	2.7%

Note: est, established.

ments increase more than networks that have a higher volume of facility-based services.

- *Provider Agreements:* The provider agreement between the health plan and the provider defines how the linkage with Medicare's RBRVS system is to be implemented. Some agreements set fees at some percentage of Medicare's fees. Others state that fees are a product of Medicare's RVUs and a contractually defined conversion factor (with or without the GPCIs). There is usually some latitude in how annual updates are implemented. If the update is expected to exceed the budget for physician services, the contract may need to be revised.

CONCLUSION

While Medicare RBRVS has become a national standard for physician fees, there are significant variations in how private payers have adapted it. These variations, when combined with the annual changes Medicare has made to the underlying components of RBRVS, may produce unintended increases in physician payments of as much as 8.5%. Private payers with RBRVS-based fee scales should analyze their entire delivery and financing systems to evaluate the overall impact of these changes on physician expenditures.

CHAPTER 18

Mini-Case Study 3:
The Economic Significance of
Resource Misallocation: A Finance
and Operations Problem in the
Women, Infants, and Children
Public Health Program

Client Flow through the Women, Infants, and Children Public Health Program*

Billie Ann Brotman, Mary Bumgarner, and Penelope Prime

CONFRONTING THE OPERATIONAL PROBLEM

The Women, Infants, and Children (WIC) Program, a federal program managed by the county boards of health, provides a mandated health service under strict federal guidelines to women and young children. In this article we analyze how a WIC clinic, located in the Atlanta metropolitan area, can serve its clientele more efficiently in an environment of constraints. We focus on achieving shorter waiting times for WIC clients through better management of the flow of clients through the clinic. We apply the peak-load framework from economics to this basic operations-research problem.

THE ENVIRONMENT

The WIC program provides nutrition counseling, limited physical examinations, and food vouchers for low-income pregnant women and for children with nutritional deficiencies who are five years old or less.

WIC represents just one part of the integrated services provided to women and children by the county clinic. Other services include inoculations, medical visits with the nurse, and a variety of social services. Providing more than one health service at the county clinic is advantageous because it reinforces good health practices, provides intervention where necessary, and is convenient for the clients. However, it also complicates the management of service provision and makes it more difficult to improve the delivery of WIC's services.

To participate in the WIC program, a certification of income and health status is required. The first step for a client is to schedule an appointment for certification with a clinic nurse. Once certified, the client is immediately eligible to receive food vouchers and can return to the clinic to pick up her vouchers for up to a year without revisiting a nurse. Vouchers may also be picked up when a client comes to the clinic for nutritional classes, which are required periodically.

From the providers' point of view, several activities directly related to the WIC program are managed simultaneously. They include the scheduling of appointments for certification, meeting previously scheduled certification appointments by the nurses, accommodating unscheduled clients who walk in

---

Source: Reprinted from B.A. Brotman, M. Bumgarner, and P. Prime, Client Flow Through the Women, Infants, and Children Public Health Program, *Journal of Health Care Finance,* Vol. 25, No. 1, pp. 72–77, © 1998, Aspen Publishers, Inc.

seeking certification, and distributing food vouchers to eligible clients. (Eligible clients include those certified by the county clinic as well as those who have been certified by Kennestone Hospital and Home Visits, and Child Health.)

In principle, the appointment system is designed to regulate these activities. In practice, several factors, none of which are within the control of the clinic staff, undermine it. First, since clients come to the clinic for other services as well, they often are delayed for their WIC appointments. Second, of those that make appointments, 40 percent–50 percent of them do not keep them, because they either arrive late or simply do not come. Understanding the obstacles many of their clients face arranging work schedules, transportation to the clinic, and child care, the clinic's management has instituted a policy of waiting 20 minutes for a client to arrive before rescheduling the appointment. Third, walk-ins are common and, according to federal guidelines, must be accommodated. In addition, the clinic has difficulty retaining qualified staff, and its physical space is limited. The end result is that women and children are often in the clinic for hours, are uncomfortable, and are unable to adequately care for their children during this time.

THE PEAK-LOAD PROBLEM

The economic problem faced by the clinic is one of demand exceeding capacity, leading to excessive wait times for the clinic's patrons as well as inefficient use of clinic nurses and clerks. The problem arises because the clinic's services are beneficial to the health of expectant mothers and children and are provided without fee to the patient. Without a price mechanism to ration demand, quantity demanded exceeds quantity supplied. This problem is not uncommon. It is encountered often in the public or quasipublic sector, when the price of the good or service does not adequately reflect the benefits of the good or service as perceived by the public.

In this case, the problem of disequilibrium between demand and supply is exacerbated by the fact that demand for the clinic's services is unpredictable. Clients often do not keep their appointments or arrive at unscheduled times. As a result, appointments may go unfilled or two or more clients may seek the same appointment time.

On the supply side, capacity constraints, coupled with a persistent lack of sufficient numbers of experienced clerks and nurses, hamper the clinic's ability to respond to unexpected demand shifts. Moreover, due to employee turnover experienced by the clinic, few employees become sufficiently skilled to work as part-time clerks during periods of peak demand.

The economic significance of the problem is one of resource misallocation. In this case, too many resources are employed in the production of WIC services. The market solution is to increase the price of the service, thereby matching demand with capacity. But since that option is not available, efficiently managing demand and supply is necessary if the amount of resources used providing WIC services is to be reduced.

Federal guidelines for the WIC program leave little maneuvering room to improve the delivery of services. For example, the clinic cannot refuse to see unscheduled walk-ins; all clients must see a nurse for certification; all clients must attend nutrition classes; and vouchers must be closely monitored. Based on the data and information provided by the clinic, we determined that the fundamental cause of the queuing problem was the time spent by clients waiting to see clerks and nurses. Our hypothesis is that the flow of traffic through the clinic can be managed more efficiently by changing the current policy of waiting 20 minutes before filling a broken appointment with a "walk-in" to a new policy of filling the appointment immediately.

METHOD

We began by collecting information on the average daily client volume, the pattern of client flow through various services, the waiting points and times, and services rendered to the clients.

The data were collected by clinic personnel during February 1994. It was recorded in a chart form throughout a day in periodic intervals and included nine items:

1. Number of clerks available
2. Number of nurses available
3. Waiting time to see clerks for walk-ins and appointments
4. Waiting time to see nurses for walk-ins and appointments
5. Total time in the clinic for walk-ins and appointments
6. Waiting time to get vouchers
7. Number of nutrition classes
8. Number of appointments met
9. Number of appointments missed.

The actual flow of traffic through the clinic is depicted in Figure 1.

Clients visit the clinic to keep an appointment with the nurse or attend a nutrition class, or as an unscheduled walk-in. All clients first see a clerk to arrange for their records to be pulled. They then check in and wait to be called to their class or appointment. At the completion of the appointment, they see a clerk to pick up vouchers. Vouchers are also distributed at the end of the nutrition classes.

The General Purpose Simulation System for personal computer (GPSS/PC) model simulates the average flow of traffic through the clinic. Estimation of traffic flow through the clinic is initiated when the client signs in and continues as the client meets with the clerks and the nurses. The model estimates the average amount of time a client spends in the clinic as well as average waiting times at each station. Clerk and nurse utilization rates are also generated assuming a variety of staffing levels. For comparison purposes, each version of the model is run with a 20-minute time lag before a late appointment is filled, and then run with a 1-minute lag.

Six versions of the model are estimated using different combinations of numbers of clerks and nurses. Model A assumes that the clinic is staffed with three nurses and three clerks, Model B with two clerks and three nurses, and Model C with two clerks and two nurses.

RESULTS

Models A, B, and C present the results of all the computer simulations.

Model A: Three Nurses and Three Clerks

A comparison of the results generated changing a 20-minute wait to a 1-minute wait show that reducing the time before an appointment is filled results in the following:

1. A decrease in the total time in the clinic for the client from 3 hours and 16 minutes to 1 hour and 11 minutes
2. A decrease in the time spent waiting for the clerk from 1 hour and 9 minutes to approximately 3 minutes
3. An increase in time spent waiting for a nurse from 3 minutes to 10 minutes
4. A decrease in the utilization of clerks from 91.6 percent to 53.2 percent
5. An increase in the utilization of nurses from 46.7 percent to 61.2 percent.

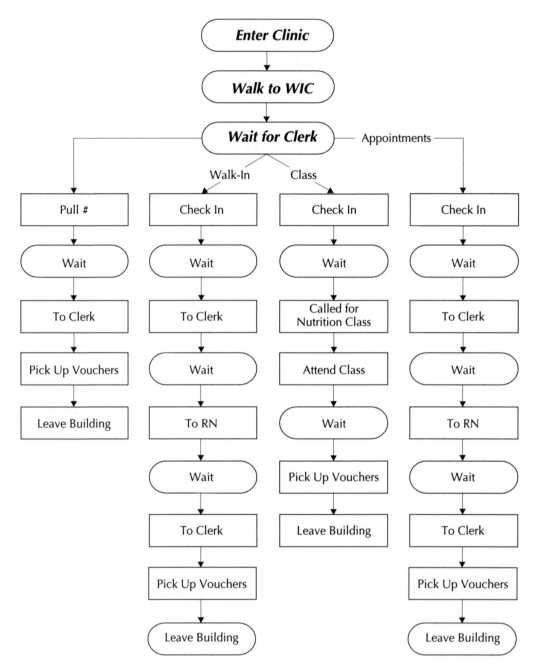

Figure 1 Traffic Flow

Model B: Three Nurses and Two Clerks

1. A decrease in the total time in the clinic for the client from 3 hours and 13 minutes to 1 hour and 27 minutes
2. A decrease in the time spent waiting for the clerk from 1 hour and 19 minutes to approximately 1 minute
3. An increase in time spent waiting for a nurse from 8 minutes to 43 minutes
4. A decrease in the utilization of clerks from 91.6 percent to 46.8 percent
5. An increase in the utilization of nurses from 51.2 percent to 73.3 percent.

Model C: Two Nurses and Two Clerks

1. A decrease in the total time in the clinic for the client from 1 hour and 50 minutes to 1 hour and 9 minutes
2. A decrease in the time spent waiting for the clerk from 19 minutes to less than 1 minute
3. A decrease in time spent waiting for a nurse from 18 minutes to 13 minutes
4. A decrease in the utilization of clerks from 76.6 percent to 30.3 percent
5. A decrease in the utilization of nurses from 64.6 percent to 53.7 percent.

•   •   •

In all three versions of the model that were estimated, the results of the simulations reveal that reducing the time before a late appointment is filled significantly decreases the time spent in the clinic by the client, on average, for all clients. Furthermore, the time spent waiting for both clerks and nurses decreases, the utilization of the clerks decreases, and the utilization of the nurses increases in two of the three estimations.

Greater decreases in waiting time occur when the clinic is staffed with three nurses and either three or two clerks. Smaller decreases occur when only two nurses and two clerks are available. This suggests that the clinic has little to no scheduling flexibility on days when it is understaffed, and a policy of filling late appointments immediately should be particularly beneficial.

The utilization of clerks and the time spent waiting for a clerk decreases in all three models when appointments are filled within one minute, and in every case but one, the utilization rate of nurses increases when appointments are filled immediately. This suggests that the flow of clients through the clinic is improved by filling appointments quickly. Utilization rates of nurses decreases only when the clinic is staffed with three nurses and three clerks. One explanation for this result is that the clinic is overstaffed with this combination of nurses and clerks. A supporting piece of evidence for this conclusion is that the change in rates of utilization for both nurses and clerks is the smallest when three of each are employed.

Another implication of these results is that if the clinic does not implement the expedited scheduling policy, it makes little difference to time spent in the clinic whether it is staffed with two nurses and two clerks or three nurses and two clerks. Both scenarios result in clients spending approximately three and a quarter hours in the clinic. With the 20-minute wait before rescheduling, the clinic must be staffed with three nurses and three clerks if the time spent in the clinic by the client is to fall below 2 hours.

In sum, our results suggest that following a policy of immediately rescheduling missed appointments reduces the misallocation of resources employed in the clinic and thus permits the clinic to respond to its clients' needs more efficiently. Although this approach cannot duplicate the increase in efficiency that could be realized through the use of a price mechanism, it does improve the overall welfare of the clinic's clients. Filling appointments immediately results in shorter wait times for all clients, so no client is made worse off by the new policy. Moreover, as the patients realize that timeliness is important, more will arrive on time, further increasing the clinic's ability to monitor demand and provide services for its clients.

Checklists

Checklist 1 Reviewing a Budget

1. Is this budget static (not adjusted for volume) or flexible (adjusted for volume during the year)?

2. Are the figures designated as fixed or variable?

3. Is the budget for a defined unit of authority?

4. Are the line items within the budget all expenses (and revenues, if applicable) that are controllable by the manager?

5. Is the format of the budget comparable with that of previous periods so that several reports over time can be compared if so desired?

6. Are actual and budget for the same period?

7. Are the figures annualized?

8. Test one line-item calculation. Is the math for the dollar difference computed correctly? Is the percentage properly computed based on a percentage of the budget figure?

Checklist 2 Building a Budget

1. What is the proposed volume for the new budget period?

2. What is the appropriate inflow (revenues) and outflow (cost of services delivered) relationship?

3. What will the appropriate dollar cost be?

    (Note: this question requires a series of assumptions about the nature of the operation for the new budget period.)

    3a. Forecast service-related workload.

    3b. Forecast non–service-related workload.

    3c. Forecast special project workload if applicable.

    3d. Coordinate assumptions for proportionate share of interdepartmental projects.

4. Will additional resources be available?

5. Will this budget accomplish the appropriate managerial objectives for the organization?

Checklist 3 Balance Sheet Review

1. What is the date on the balance sheet?

2. Are there large discrepancies in balances between the prior year and the current year?

3. Did total assets increase over the prior year?

4. Did current assets increase, decrease, or stay about the same?

5. Did current liabilities increase, decrease, or stay about the same?

6. Did land, plant, and equipment increase or decrease significantly over the prior year?

7. Did long-term debt increase or decrease significantly over the prior year?

Checklist 4 Review of the Statement of Revenue and Expense

1. What is the period reported on the statement of revenue and expense?

2. Is it one year or a shorter period? If it is a shorter period, why is that?

3. Are there large discrepancies in balances between the prior year operations and the current year operations?

4. Did total operating revenue increase over the prior year?

5. Did total operating expenses increase, decrease, or stay about the same? Is any particular line item unusually large or small?

6. Did income from operations increase, decrease, or stay about the same?

7. Are there unusual nonoperating gains or losses?

8. Did the current year result in an excess of revenue over expense? Is it as much as that of the prior year?

9. Did long-term debt increase or decrease significantly over the prior year?

Web-Based Learning Tools

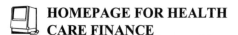

HOMEPAGE FOR HEALTH CARE FINANCE

Basic tools for the Nonfinancial Manager has its own homepage on Aspen's web site. The homepage contains resources for both instructors and students. The site can be accessed using the following URL: http://www.aspenpublishers.com/books/hcfinance.html.

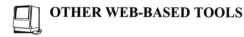

OTHER WEB-BASED TOOLS

Users who prefer to use a business analyst calculator (as opposed to computer spreadsheets) can refer to the Texas Instruments site at www.ti.com/calc. A guide book for operating the BAII Plus can be found there. Readers who desire self-study continuing professional education credits may go to www.helix-cpe.com.

Notes

Chapter 1

1. C. S. George, Jr., *The History of Management Thought*, 2nd ed. (Englewood Cliffs, NJ: Prentice Hall, 1972), 1–27.
2. C. S. George Jr., *The History of Management Thought*, 2nd ed. (Englewood Cliffs, NJ: Prentice Hall, 1972), 87.

Chapter 2

1. S. Williamson et al., *Fundamentals of Strategic Planning for Healthcare Organizations* (New York: The Haworth Press, 1997).

Chapter 3

1. J. J. Baker, *Activity-Based Costing and Activity-Based Management for Health Care* (Gaithersburg, MD: Aspen Publishers, Inc., 1998).
2. L. V. Seawell, *Chart of Accounts for Hospitals* (Chicago: Probus Publishing Company, 1994).

Chapter 4

1. Texas Medical Association, American Medical Association, Texas Medical Foundation, and Texas Osteopathic Medical Association, *A Guide to Forming Physician-Directed Managed Care Networks* (Austin, TX: Texas Medical Association, 1994), 3.
2. Health Care Financing Administration, *Health Care Financing Review: Medicare and Medicaid Statistical Supplement* (Baltimore, MD: U.S. Department of Health and Human Services, 1997), 8.
3. Health Care Financing Administration, *Health Care Financing Review: Medicare and Medicaid Statistical Supplement* (Baltimore, MD: U.S. Department of Health and Human Services, 1997), 9.

4. D. I. Samuels, *Capitation: New Opportunities in Healthcare Delivery* (Chicago: Irwin Professional Publishing, 1996), 20–21.
5. D. E. Goldstein, *Alliances: Strategies for Building Integrated Delivery Systems* (Gaithersburg, MD: Aspen Publishers, Inc., 1995), 283; and Texas Medical Association, American Medical Association, Texas Medical Foundation, and Texas Osteopathic Medical Association, *A Guide to Forming Physician-Directed Managed Care Networks* (Austin, TX: Texas Medical Association, 1994), 4–6.
6. C. Horngren et al., *Cost Accounting: A Managerial Emphasis*, 9th ed. (Englewood Cliffs, NJ: Prentice Hall, 1998), 116.
7. A. Sharpe and G. Jaffe, "Columbia/HCA Plans for More Big Changes in Health-Care World," *The Wall Street Journal*, 28 May 1997, A8.

Chapter 5

1. S. A. Finkler, *Essentials of Cost Accounting for Health Care Organizations*, 2nd ed. (Gaithersburg, MD: Aspen Publishers, Inc., 1999).
2. G. F. Longshore, "Service-Line Management/Bottom-Line Management," *Journal of Health Care Finance* 24, no. 4 (1998): 72–79.

Chapter 6

1. C. Horngren et al., *Cost Accounting: A Managerial Emphasis*, 9th ed. (Englewood Cliffs, NJ: Prentice Hall, 1998), 70.
2. J. J. Baker, *Activity-Based Costing and Activity-Based Management for Health Care* (Gaithersburg, MD: Aspen Publishers, Inc., 1998).

3. D. A. West, T. D. West, and P.J. Malone, "Managing Capital and Administrative (Indirect) Costs to Achieve Strategic Objectives: The Dialysis Clinic versus the Outpatient Clinic," *Journal of Health Care Finance* 25 no. 2 (1998): 20–34.

Chapter 7

1. J. J. Baker, *Activity-Based Costing and Activity-Based Management for Health Care* (Gaithersburg, MD: Aspen Publishers, Inc., 1998).

2. C. Horngren et al., *Cost Accounting: A Managerial Emphasis*, 9th ed. (Englewood Cliffs, NJ: Prentice Hall, 1998).

Chapter 8

1. J. J. Baker, *Prospective Payment for Long-Term Care: An Annual Guide* (Gaithersburg, MD: Aspen Publishers, Inc., 1999).

2. J. J. Baker, *Prospective Payment for Long-Term Care: An Annual Guide* (Gaithersburg, MD: Aspen Publishers, Inc., 1999).

Chapter 9

1. B. A. Brotman, M. Bumgarner, and P. Prime, "Client Flow through the Women, Infants and Children Public Health Program," *Journal of Health Care Finance* 25, no. 1 (1998): 72–77.

Chapter 10

1. W. O. Cleverly, *Essentials of Health Care Finance,* 4th ed. (Gaithersburg, MD: Aspen Publishers, Inc., 1997).

2. C. Horngren et al., *Cost Accounting: A Managerial Emphasis*, 9th ed. (Englewood Cliffs, NJ: Prentice Hall, 1998), 227.

3. C. Horngren et al., *Cost Accounting: A Managerial Emphasis*, 9th ed. (Englewood Cliffs, NJ: Prentice Hall, 1998), 228.

4. J. R. Pearson et al., *The Flexible Budget Process—A Tool for Cost Containment, A. J. C. P.* 84, no. 2 (1985): 202-208.

5. S. A. Finkler, "Flexible Budget Variance Analysis Extended to Patient Acuity and DRGs," *Health Care Management Review* 10, no. 4 (1985): 21–34.

Chapter 11

1. S. Williamson et al., *Fundamentals of Strategic Planning for Healthcare Organizations* (New York: The Haworth Press, 1997).

Chapter 12

1. S. A. Finkler, *Essentials of Cost Accounting for Health Care Organizations*, 2nd ed. (Gaithersburg, MD: Aspen Publishers, Inc., 1999).

Glossary

Accounting System: Records the evidence that some event has occurred in the health care financial system.

Accrual Basis Accounting: Revenue is recorded when it is earned, not when payment is received. Expenses are recorded when they are incurred, not when they are paid. The opposite of accrual basis is cash basis accounting.

Balance Sheet: One of the four basic financial statements. Generally speaking, the balance sheet records what an organization owns, what it owes, and what it is worth at a particular point in time.

Benchmarking: The continuous process of measuring products, services, and activities against the best levels of performance. Such best levels may be found inside the organization or outside it.

Breakeven Point: The point when the contribution margin (i.e., net revenues less variable costs) equals the fixed costs.

Budget: The organization-wide instrument through which activities are quantified in financial terms.

Case Mix Adjusted: A performance measure that has been adjusted for the acuity level of the patient and, presumably, the resource level required to provide care.

Cash Basis Accounting: A transaction does not enter the books until cash is either received or paid out. The opposite of cash basis is accrual basis accounting.

Chart of Accounts: Maps out account titles in a uniform manner through a method of numeric coding.

Common Sizing: A process of converting dollar amounts to percentages in order to put information on the same relative basis. Also known as *vertical analysis*.

Contribution Margin: So called because it contributes to fixed costs and to profits. Computed as net revenues less variable costs.

Controllable Expenses: Subject to a manager's own decision making, and thus *controllable*.

Controlling: Making sure that each area of the organization is following the plans that have been established.

Cost: The amount of cash expended (or property transferred, services performed, or liability incurred) in consideration of goods or services received or to be received.

Cost-Profit-Volume (CPV): The method of illustrating the breakeven point, whereby the three elements of cost, profit, and volume are accounted for within the computation.

Cost Object: Any unit for which a separate cost measurement is desired.

Current Ratio: A liquidity ratio considered to be a measure of short-term, debt-paying ability. Computed by dividing current assets by current liabilities.

Days Cash on Hand Ratio: A liquidity ratio that indicates the number of days of operating expenses represented in the amount of unrestricted cash on hand. Computed by dividing unrestricted cash and cash equivalents by the cash operating expenses divided by number of days in the period.

Days Receivables Ratio: A liquidity ratio that represents the number of days in receivables. Computed by dividing net receivables by net credit revenues divided by number of days in the period.

Debt Service Coverage Ratio: A solvency ratio universally used in credit analysis to measure ability to pay debt service. Computed by dividing change in unrestricted net assets (net income) plus interest, depreciation, and amortization by maximum annual debt service.

Decision Making: Making choices among available alternatives.

Diagnoses: A common method of grouping health care expenses for purposes of planning and control. Such a grouping may be by major diagnostic categories (MDCs) or by diagnosis-related groups (DRGs).

Direct Cost: These costs are incurred for the sole benefit of a particular operating unit. They can therefore be specifically associated with a particular unit or department or patient. Laboratory tests are an example of a direct cost.

Discounted Fee-for-Service: The provider of services is paid according to an agreed upon contracted discount and after the service is delivered.

Expenses: Actual or expected cash outflows incurred in the course of doing business. Expenses are the costs that relate to the earning of revenue. An example is salary expense for labor performed.

Expired Costs: Costs that are used up in the current period and are matched against current revenues.

Fee-for-Service: The provider of services is paid according to the service performed, after the service is delivered.

Financial Accounting: Is generally for outside, or third party, use and thus emphasizes external reporting.

Fixed Cost: Those costs that do not vary in total when activity levels or volume of operations change. Rent expense is an example of fixed cost.

Flexible Budget: A budget based on a range of activity or volume. The flexible budget is adjusted, or flexed (thus "flexible"), to the actual level of output achieved or expected to be achieved during the budget period.

Forecasts: Information used for purposes of planning for the future. Forecasts can be short-range, intermediate-range, or long-range.

Full Time Equivalents (FTEs): A measure to express the equivalent of an employee (annualized) or a position (staffed) for the full time required.

General Ledger: A document in which all transactions for the period reside.

General Services Expenses: This type of expense provides services necessary to maintain the patient, but the service is not directly related to patient care. Examples of general services expenses are laundry and dietary.

Horizontal Analysis: The process of comparing and analyzing figures over several time periods. Also known as *trend analysis*.

Indirect Cost: These costs are incurred on behalf of the overall operation and therefore cannot be associated with the provision of specific health services. The finance office is an example of an indirect cost. Also known as *joint costs*.

Information System: Gathers the evidence that some event has occurred in the health care financial system.

Internal Rate of Return: A return on investment method, defined as the rate of interest that discounts future net inflows (from the proposed investment) down to the amount invested.

Joint Cost: These costs are incurred on behalf of the overall operation and therefore cannot be associated with the provision of specific health services. The finance office is an example of a joint cost. Also known as *indirect costs*.

Liabilities to Fund Balance Ratio: A solvency ratio used as a quick indicator of debt load. Computed by dividing total liabilities by unrestricted net assets. Also known as *debt to net worth ratio*.

Liquidity Ratios: Ratios that reflect the ability of the organization to meet its current obligations. Liquidity ratios are measures of short-term sufficiency.

Managed Care: A means of providing health care services within a network of health care providers. The central concept is coordination of all health care services for an individual.

Managerial Accounting: Is generally for inside, or internal, use and thus emphasizes information useful for managerial employees.

Medicaid Program: A federal and state matching entitlement program intended to provide medical assistance to eligible needy individuals and families. The program was established under Title XIX of the Social Security Act.

Medicare Program: A federal health insurance program for the aged (and, in certain instances, for the disabled) intended to complement other federal benefits. The program was established under Title XVIII of the Social Security Act.

Mixed Cost: Those costs that contain an element of variable cost and an element of fixed cost.

Non-Controllable Expenses: Outside the manager's power to make decisions.

Nonproductive Time: Paid-for time when the employee is not on duty; that is, not producing. Paid-for vacation days and holidays are examples of nonproductive time.

Nonprofit Organization: Indicates the taxable status of the organization. A nonprofit (or voluntary) organization is exempt from paying income taxes. See also *voluntary*.

Operating Margin: A profitability ratio generally expressed as a percentage, the operating margin is a multipurpose measure. It is used for a number of managerial purposes and also sometimes enters into credit analysis. Computed by dividing operating income (loss) by total operating revenues.

Operations Expenses: This type of expense provides service directly related to patient care. Examples of operations expenses are radiology expense and drug expense.

Organization Chart: Indicates the formal lines of communication and reporting and how responsibility is assigned to managers.

Organizing: Deciding how to use the resources of the organization to most effectively carry out the plans that have been established.

Original Records: Provide evidence that some event has occurred in the health care financial system.

Pareto Analysis: An analytical tool employing the Pareto principle, also known as the 80/20 rule. For example, the Pareto principle states that 80 percent of an organization's problems are caused by 20 percent of the possible causes.

Payback Period: The length of time required for the cash coming in from an investment to equal the amount of cash originally spent when the investment was acquired.

Payer Mix: The proportion of revenues realized from different types of payers. A measure often included in the profile of a health care organization.

Performance Measures: Measures that compare and quantify performance. Performance measures may be financial, nonfinancial, or a combination of both types.

Period Cost: For purposes of health care businesses, period cost is necessary to support the existence of the organization itself, rather than actual delivery of a service. Period costs are matched with revenue on the basis of the period during which the cost is incurred. The term originated with the manufacturing industry.

Planning: Identifying objectives of the organization and identifying the steps required to accomplish the objectives.

Present Value Analysis: A concept based on the time value of money. The value of a dollar today is more than the value of a dollar in the future.

Procedures: A common method of grouping health care expenses for purposes of planning and control. Such a grouping will generally be by Physicians' Current Procedural Terminology, or CPT, codes, which list descriptive terms and identifying codes for medical services and procedures performed.

Product Cost: For purposes of health care businesses, product cost is necessary to actually deliver the service. The term originated with the manufacturing industry.

Productive Time: Equates to the employee's net hours on duty when performing the functions in his or her job description.

Profit Center: Makes a manager responsible for both the revenue/volume (inflow) side and the expense (outflow) side of a department, division, unit, or program. Also known as a *responsibility center*.

Profitability Ratios: Ratios that reflect the ability of the organization to operate with an excess of operating revenue over operating expense.

Profit-Oriented Organization: Indicates the taxable status of the organization. A profit-oriented (or proprietary) organization is responsible for paying income taxes.

Profit-Volume (PV) Ratio: The contribution margin (i.e., net revenues less variable costs) expressed as a percentage of net revenue.

Quartiles: A distribution into four classes, each of which contains one-quarter of the whole; any one of the four classes is a quartile.

Quick Ratio: A liquidity ratio considered to be the most severe test of short-term debt-paying ability (even more severe than the current ratio). Computed by dividing cash and cash equivalents plus net receivables by current liabilities. Also known as the *acid-test ratio*.

Proprietary Organization: Indicates the taxable status of the organization. A proprietary (or profit-oriented) organization is responsible for paying income taxes. See also *profit-oriented.*

Reporting System: Produces reports of an event's effect in the health care financial system.

Responsibility Centers: Makes a manager responsible for both the revenue/volume (inflow) side and the expense (outflow) side of a department, division, unit, or program. Also known as a *profit center.*

Return on Total Assets: A profitability ratio generally expressed as a percentage, this is a broad measure of profitability in common use. Computed by dividing earnings before interest and taxes, or EBIT, by total assets. This ratio is known by its acronym EBIT in credit analysis circles.

Revenue: Actual or expected cash inflows due to the organization's major business. Revenues are amounts earned in the course of doing business. In the case of health care, revenues are mostly earned by rendering services to patients.

Semi-Fixed Cost: Those costs that stay fixed for a time when activity levels or volume of operations change; rises will occur, but not in direct proportion.

Semi-Variable Cost: Those costs that vary when activity levels or volume of operations change, but not in direct proportion. A supervisor's salary is an example of a semi-variable cost.

Solvency Ratios: Ratios that reflect the ability of the organization to pay the annual interest and principal obligations on its long-term debt. These ratios determine ability to "be solvent."

Staffing: A term which means the assigning of staff to fill scheduled positions.

Statement of Cash Flows: One of the four basic statements, this statement reports the current period cash flow by taking the accrual basis statements and converting them to an effective cash flow. This is accomplished by a series of reconciling adjustments that account for the non-cash amounts.

Statement of Fund Balance/Net Worth: One of the four basic statements, this statement reports the excess of revenue over expenses (or vice-versa) for the period as the excess flows into equity (or reduces equity, in the case of a loss for the period).

Statement of Revenue and Expense: One of the four basic financial statements, this statement reports the inflow of revenue and the outflow of expense over a stated period of time. The net result is also reported, either as excess of revenue over expense, or, in the case of a loss for the period, excess of expense over revenue.

Static Budget: A budget based on a single level of operations, or volume. Once approved and finalized, the single level of operations (volume) is never adjusted; thus the budget is "static" or unchanging.

Subsidiary Journals: Documents which contain specific sets of transactions and which support the general ledger.

Subsidiary Reports: Reports which support, and thus are subsidiary to, the four major financial statements.

Support Services Expenses: This type of expense provides support to both general services expenses and to operations expenses. It is necessary for support, but it is neither directly related to patient care nor is it a service necessary to maintain the patient. Examples of support services are insurance and payroll taxes.

Time Value of Money: The present value concept, which is that the value of a dollar today is more than the value of a dollar in the future.

Three-Variance Method: A method of variance analysis that compares volume variance to use (or quantity) variance and to spending (or price) variance.

Trend Analysis: The process of comparing and analyzing figures over several time periods. Also known as *horizontal analysis*.

Trial Balance: A document used to balance the general ledger accounts and to produce financial statements.

Two-Variance Method: A method of variance analysis that compares volume variance to budgeted costs (defined as standard hours for actual production).

Unadjusted Rate of Return: An unsophisticated return on investment method, the answer for which is an estimate containing no precision.

Unexpired Costs: Costs that are not yet used up and will be matched against future revenues.

Variable Cost: Those costs that vary in direct proportion to changes in activity levels of volume of operations. Food for meal preparation is an example of variable cost.

Variance Analysis: A variance is the difference between standard and actual prices and quantities. Variance analysis analyzes these differences.

Vertical Analysis: A process of converting dollar amounts to percentages to put information on the same relative basis. Also known as *common sizing*.

Voluntary Organization: Indicates the taxable status of the organization. A voluntary (or nonprofit) organization is exempt from paying income taxes.

Examples and Exercises, Supplemental Material, and Solutions

The following examples and exercises include examples, practice exercises, and assignment exercises. Solutions to the practice exercises are found at the end of this section. Exercises are designated by chapter number.

EXAMPLES AND EXERCISES

CHAPTER 2

Assignment Exercise 2–1

Review the chapter text about types of organizations and examine the list in Exhibit 2–1.

Required

1. Obtain listings of health care organizations from the yellow pages of a telephone book.
2. Set up a work sheet listing the classifications of organizations found in Exhibit 2–1.
3. Enter the organizations you found in the yellow pages onto the work sheet.
4. For each organization indicate the type of organization.
5. If some cannot be identified by type, comment on what you would expect them to be; that is, proprietary, voluntary, or government owned.

Assignment Exercise 2–2

Review the chapter text about organization charts. Also examine the organization charts appearing in Figures 2–1 and 2–2.

Required

1. Refer to the Metropolis Health System (MHS) case study appearing in Chapter 15. Read about the various types of services offered by MHS.

2. The MHS organization chart has seven major areas of responsibility, each headed by a senior vice president. Select one of the seven areas and design additional levels of detail that indicate the managers. If you have considerable detail you may choose one department (such as ambulatory operations) instead of the entire area of responsibility for that senior vice president.
3. Do you believe your design of the detailed organization chart indicates centralized or decentralized lines of authority for decision making? Can you explain your approach in one to two sentences?

CHAPTER 3

Assignment Exercise 3–1: Health System Flowsheets

Review the chapter text about information flow and Figures 3–2 and 3–3.

Required

1. Find an information flowsheet from a health care organization. It can be from a published source or from an actual organization.
2. Based on this flowsheet, comment on what the structure of the organization's information system appears to be.
3. If you were a manager (at this organization), would you want to change the structure? If so, why? If not, why not?

Assignment Exercise 3–2: Chart of Accounts

Review the chapter text about the chart of accounts and how it is a map of the company elements. Also review Exhibits 3–1, 3–2, and 3–3.

Required

1. Find an excerpt from a health care organization's chart of accounts. It can be from a published source or from an actual organization.
2. Based on this chart of accounts excerpt, comment on what the structure of the organization's reporting system appears to be.
3. If you were a manager (at this organization), would you want to change the system? If so, why? If not, why not?

CHAPTER 4

Example 4A: Contractual Allowances

Contractual allowances represent the difference between the full established rate and the agreed-upon contractual rate that will be paid. An example was given in the text of Chapter 4 by which the hospital's full established rate for a certain procedure is $100, but Giant Health Plan has negotiated a managed care contract whereby the plan pays only $90 for that procedure. The contractual allowance is $10 ($100 less $90 = $10). Assume instead that Near-By Health Plan has negotiated its own managed care contract whereby this plan pays $95 for that procedure. In this case the contractual allowance is $5 ($100 less $95 = $5).

Assignment Exercise 4–1: Contractual Allowances

Physician Office Revenue for Visit Code 99214 has a full established rate of $72.00. Of ten different payers, there are nine different contracted rates, as follows:

Payer	Contracted Rate
FHP	$35.70
HPHP	58.85
MC	54.90
UND	60.40
CCN	70.20
MO	70.75
CGN	10.00
PRU	54.90
PHCS	50.00
ANA	45.00

Rates for illustration only.

Required

1. Set up a work sheet with four columns: *Payer, Full Rate, Contracted Rate,* and *Contractual Allowance.*
2. For each payer, enter the full rate and the contracted rate.
3. For each payer, compute the contractual allowance.

The first payer has been computed below:

Payer	Full Rate	(less)	Contracted Rate	=	Contractual Allowance
FHP	$72.00		$35.70		$36.30

Example 4B: Revenue Sources and Grouping Revenue

Sources of health care revenue are often grouped by payer. Thus services might be grouped as follows:

Revenue from the Medicare Program (payer = Medicare)
Revenue from the Medicaid Program (payer = Medicaid)
Revenue from Blue Cross Blue Shield (payer = Commercial Insurance)
or
Revenue from Blue Cross Blue Shield (payer = Managed Care Contract)

Assignment Exercise 4–2: Revenue Sources and Grouping Revenue

The Metropolis Health System has revenue sources from operations, donations, and interest income. The revenue from operations is primarily received for services. MHS groups its revenue first by cost center. Within each cost center the services revenue is then grouped by payer.

Required

1. Set up a work sheet with individual columns across the top for six revenue sources (payers): *Medicare, Medicaid, Other Public Programs, Patients, Commercial Insurance,* and *Managed Care Contracts.*
2. Certain situations concerning the Intensive Care Unit and the Laboratory are described below.

   Set up six vertical line items on your work sheet, numbered (1) through (6). Six situations are described below. For each of the six situations, indicate its number (1 through 6) and enter the appropriate cost center (either Intensive Care Unit or Laboratory). Then place an X in the column(s) that represents the correct revenue source(s) for the item. The six situations are as follows:

   (1) ICU stay billed to employee's insurance program.
   (2) Lab test paid for by an individual.
   (3) Pathology work performed for the state.
   (4) ICU stay billed to member's health plan.
   (5) ICU stay billed for Medicare beneficiary.
   (6) Series of allergy tests run for eligible Medicaid beneficiary.

Headings for your work sheet:

Medicare	Medicaid	Other Public Programs	Patients	Commercial Insurance	Managed Care Contracts
(1)					
(2)					
(3)					
(4)					
(5)					
(6)					

CHAPTER 5

Example 5A: Grouping Expenses by Cost Center

Cost centers are one method of grouping expenses. For example, a nursing home may consider the Admitting Department as a cost center. In that case the expenses grouped under the Admitting Department cost center may include:

- Administrative and Clerical Salaries
- Admitting Supplies
- Dues
- Periodicals and Books

- Employee Education
- Purchased Maintenance

Practice Exercise 5–I: Grouping Expenses by Cost Center

The Metropolis Health System groups expenses for the Intensive Care Unit into its own cost center. Laboratory expenses and Laundry expenses are likewise grouped into their own cost centers.

Required

1. Set up a work sheet with individual columns across the top for the three cost centers: *Intensive Care Unit*, *Laboratory*, and *Laundry*.
2. Indicate the appropriate cost center for each of the following expenses:
   - Drugs Requisitioned
   - Pathology Supplies
   - Detergents and Bleach
   - Nursing Salaries
   - Clerical Salaries
   - Uniforms (for Laundry Aides)
   - Repairs (parts for microscopes)
   (Hint: One of the expenses will apply to more than one cost center.)

Headings for your worksheet:

Intensive Care Unit   *Laboratory*   *Laundry*

Assignment Exercise 5–1: Grouping Expenses by Cost Center

The Metropolis Health System's Rehabilitation and Wellness Center offers outpatient therapy and return-to-work services plus cardiac and pulmonary rehabilitation to get people back to a normal way of living. The Rehabilitation and Wellness Center expenses include the following:

- Nursing Salaries
- Physical Therapist Salaries
- Occupational Therapist Salaries
- Cardiac Rehab Salaries
- Pulmonary Rehab Salaries
- Patient Education Coordinator Salary
- Nursing Supplies
- Physical Therapist Supplies
- Occupational Therapist Supplies
- Cardiac Rehab Supplies
- Pulmonary Rehab Supplies
- Training Supplies
- Clerical Office Supplies
- Employee Education

Required

1. Decide how many cost centers should be used for the above expenses at the Center.
2. Set up a work sheet with individual columns across the top for the cost centers you have chosen.

3. For each of the expenses listed above, indicate to which of your cost centers it should be assigned.

Example 5B

Study the chapter text concerning grouping expenses by diagnoses and procedures. Refer to Exhibits 5–3 and 5–4 (about Major Diagnostic Categories), Exhibit 5–5 (about DRGs and MDCs), and Table 5–1 (about Procedure Codes) for examples of different ways to group expenses by diagnoses and procedures.

Assignment Exercise 5–2

Required

Find a listing of expenses by diagnosis or by procedure. The source of the list can be internal (within a health care facility of some type) or external (such as a published article, report, or survey). Comment upon whether you believe the expense grouping used is appropriate. Would you have grouped the expenses in another way?

CHAPTER 6

Example 6A: Direct and Indirect Costs

Review the chapter text regarding direct and indirect costs. In particular review the example of freestanding dialysis center direct costs (Exhibit 6–1) and indirect costs (Exhibit 6–2). Remember that indirect costs are shared and are sometimes called joint costs or common costs. Because such costs are shared they must be allocated. Also, remember that one test of a direct cost is to ask: "If the operating unit (such as a department) did not exist, would this cost not be in existence?"

Practice Exercise 6–I: Identifying Direct and Indirect Costs

Make a worksheet with two columns labeled: *Direct Cost* and *Indirect Cost*. Place each of the following items in the appropriate column:

- Managed care marketing expense
- Real estate taxes
- Liability insurance
- Clinic telephone expense
- Utilities (for the entire facility)
- Emergency room medical supplies

Assignment Exercise 6–1: Allocating Indirect Costs

Study Table 6–1, Example of Radiology Departments Direct and Indirect Cost Totals, and Table 6–2, Example of Indirect Costs Allocated to Radiology Departments, and review the chapter text describing how the indirect cost is allocated. This assignment will change the allocation bases: A) Volumes, B) Direct Costs, and C) Number of Films.

Required

1. Compute the costs allocated to cost centers #557, 558, 559, 560, and 561 using the new allocation bases shown below. Use a worksheet replicating the set up in Table 6–2. Total the new results.

   The new allocation bases are:

A) Volumes	120,000	130,000	70,000	110,000	70,000	500,000
B) Direct costs	$1,100,000	$700,000	$1,300,000	$1,600,000	$1,300,000	$6,000,000
C) No. of films	400,000	20,000	55,000	25,000	20,000	520,000

2. Using a worksheet replicating the set up in Table 6–1, enter the new direct cost and the new totals for indirect costs resulting from your work. Total the new results.

Practice Exercise 6–II: Responsibility Centers

The Metropolis Health System has one Director who supervises the areas of Security, Communications, and Ambulance Services. This Director also supervises the Medical Records relevant to Ambulance Services, the educational training for Security and Ambulance Services personnel, and the human resources for Security, Communications, and Ambulance Services personnel.

Required

Of the duties and services described above, all of which are supervised by one Director, which areas should be Responsibility Centers and which areas should be Support Centers? Draw them in a visual and indicate the reporting requirements.

Assignment Exercise 6–2: Responsibility Centers

Choose among the Physician's Practice in Mini-Case Study #2, the Clinic in Mini-Case Study #3, or Continuing Care Retirement Center in Mini-Case Study #1. Designate the Responsibility Centers and the Support Centers for the organization selected. Prepare a rationale for the structure you have designed.

CHAPTER 7

Example 7A: Fixed, Variable, and Semivariable Distinction

Review the chapter text for the distinction between fixed, variable, and semivariable costs. Pay particular attention to the accompanying Figures 7–1, 7–2, 7–3, 7–4, and 7–5.

Practice Exercise 7–I: Analyzing Mixed Costs

The Metropolis Health System has a system-wide training course for nurse aides. The course requires a packet of materials that MHS calls the *training pack*. Due to turnover and because the course is system-wide, there is a monthly demand for new packs. In addition the local community college also obtains the training packs used in their credit courses from MHS.

The Education Coordinator needs to know how much of the cost is fixed and how much of the cost is variable for these training packs. She decides to use the high-low method of computation.

Required

Using the monthly utilization information presented below, find the fixed and variable portion of costs through the high-low method.

Month	Number of Training Packs	Cost
January	1,000	$6,200
February	200	1,820
March	250	2,350
April	400	3,440
May	700	4,900
June	300	2,730
July	150	1,470
August	100	1,010
September	1,100	7,150
October	300	2,850
November	250	2,300
December	100	1,010

Assignment Exercise 7–1: Analyzing Mixed Costs

The Education Coordinator decides that the Community College packs may be unduly influencing the high-low computation. She decides to re-run the results omitting the Community College volume.

Required

1. Using the monthly utilization information presented below, and omitting the Community College training packs, find the fixed and variable portion of costs through the high-

low method. Note that the college only acquires packs in three months of the year: January, May, and September. These dates coincide with the start dates of their semesters and summer school.

2. The reason the Education Coordinator needs to know how much of the cost is fixed is because she is supposed to collect the appropriate variable cost from the Community College for their packs. For her purposes, which computation do you believe is better? Why?

Month	Total Number of Training Packs	Total Cost	Community College Number Packs	Community College Cost
January	1,000	$6,200	200	$1,240
February	200	1,820		
March	250	2,350		
April	400	3,440		
May	700	4,900	300	2,100
June	300	2,730		
July	150	1,470		
August	100	1,010		
September	1,100	7,150	300	1,950
October	300	2,850		
November	250	2,300		
December	100	1,010		

Example 7B: Contribution Margin

Computation of a contribution margin is simplified if the fixed and variable expense has already been determined. Examine Table 7–1, which contains Operating Room Fixed and Variable Costs. We can see that the total costs are $1,217,756. Of this amount, $600,822 is designated as variable cost and $616,934 is designated as fixed ($529,556 + $87,378 = $616,934). For purposes of our example, assume the Operating Room revenue amounts to $1,260,000. The contribution margin is computed as follows:

	Amount
Revenue	$1,260,000
Less Variable Cost	(600,822)
Contribution Margin	$ 659,178

Thus $659,178 is available to contribute to fixed costs and to profit. (In this example fixed costs amount to $616,934, so there is an amount left to contribute toward profit.)

Practice Exercise 7–II: Calculating the Contribution Margin

Greenside Clinic has revenue totaling $3,500,000. The clinic has costs totaling $3,450,000. Of this amount, 40 percent is variable cost and 60 percent is fixed cost.

Required

Compute the contribution margin for Greenside Clinic.

Assignment Exercise 7–2: Calculating the Contribution Margin

The Mental Health program for the Community Center has just completed its fiscal year end. The Program Director determines that his program has revenue for the year of $1,210,000. He believes his variable expense amounts to $205,000 and he knows his fixed expense amounts to $1,100,000.

Required

1. Compute the contribution margin for the Community Center Mental Health program.
2. What does the result tell you about the program?

Example 7C: Cost-Volume-Profit (CVP) Ratio and Profit-Volume (PV) Ratio

Closely review the examples of ratio calculations in the chapter text. Also note that examples are presented in visuals as well as text.

Practice Exercise 7–III: Calculating the PV Ratio

The Profit-Volume (PV) Ratio is also known as the Contribution Margin (CM) Ratio. Use the same assumptions for the Community Center Mental Health Program. In addition to the contribution margin figures already computed, now compute the PV Ratio (also known as CM Ratio).

Assignment Exercise 7–3: Calculating the PV Ratio and the CVP Ratio

Use the same assumptions for the Greenside Clinic. One more assumption will be added: the Clinic had 35,000 visits.

Required

1. In addition to the contribution margin figures already computed, now compute the PV Ratio (also known as CM Ratio).
2. Add another column to your worksheet and compute the clinic's per-visit revenue and costs.
3. Create a Cost-Volume-Profit chart. Refer to the chapter text along with Figure 7–6.

CHAPTER 8

Example 8A

Review the chapter text about annualizing positions. In particular review Exhibit 8–2, which contains the annualizing calculations.

Practice Exercise 8–I: FTEs To Annualize Staffing

The office manager for a physicians' group affiliated with Metropolis Health System is working on her budget for next year. She wants to annualize her staffing plan. To do so she needs to convert her staff's net paid days worked to a factor. Their office is open and staffed seven days a week, per their agreement with two managed care plans.

The office manager has the MHS work sheet, which shows 9 holidays, 7 sick days, 15 vacation days, and 3 education days, equaling 34 paid days per year not worked. The physicians' group allows 8 holidays, 5 sick days, and 1 education day. An employee must work one full year to earn 5 vacation days. An employee must have worked full time for three full years before earning 10 annual vacation days. Because the turnover is so high, nobody on staff has earned more than 5 vacation days.

Required

1. Compute Net Paid Days Worked for a full-time employee in the physicians' group.
2. Convert Net Paid Days Worked to a factor so the office manager can annualize her staffing plan.

Assignment Exercise 8–1: FTEs To Annualize Staffing

The Metropolis Health System managers are also working on their budgets for next year. Each manager must annualize his or her staffing plan, and thus must convert staff net paid days worked to a factor. Each manager has the MHS work sheet, which shows 9 holidays, 7 sick days, 15 vacation days, and 3 education days, equaling 34 paid days per year not worked.

The Laboratory is fully staffed seven days per week and the 34 paid days per year not worked is applicable for the lab. The Medical Records department is also fully staffed seven days per week. However, Medical Records is an outsourced department so the employee benefits are somewhat different. The Medical Records employees receive 9 holidays plus 21 personal leave days which can be used for any purpose.

Required

1. Compute Net Paid Days Worked for a full-time employee in the Laboratory and in Medical Records.
2. Convert Net Paid Days Worked to a factor for the Laboratory and for Medical Records so these MHS managers can annualize their staffing plans.

Example 8B

Review the chapter text about staffing requirements to fill a position. In particular review Exhibit 8–4, which contains (at the bottom of the exhibit) the staffing calculations. Remember this method uses a basic work week as the standard.

Practice Exercise 8–II: FTEs To Fill a Position

Metropolis Health System (MHS) uses a basic work week of 40 hours throughout the system. Thus one full-time employee works 40 hours per week. MHS also uses a standard 24-hour scheduling system of three 8-hour shifts. The Admissions manager needs to compute the staffing requirements to fill his departmental positions. He has more than one Admissions office staffed within the system. The West Admissions office typically has two Admissions officers on duty during the day shift, one Admissions officer on duty during the evening shift, and one Admissions officer on duty during the night shift. The day shift also has one clerical person on duty. Staffing is identical for all seven days of the week.

Required

1. Set up a staffing requirements worksheet, using the format in Exhibit 8–4.
2. Compute the number of FTEs required to fill the Admissions officer position and the clerical position at the West Admissions office.

Assignment Exercise 8–2: FTEs To Fill a Position

Metropolis Health System (MHS) uses a basic work week of 40 hours throughout the system. Thus one full-time employee works 40 hours per week. MHS also uses a standard 24-hour scheduling system of three 8-hour shifts. The Director of Nursing needs to compute the staffing requirements to fill the Operating Room positions. Since MHS is a trauma center the OR is staffed 24 hours a day, 7 days a week. At present, staffing is identical for all seven days of the week, although the Director of Nursing is questioning the efficiency of this method.

The Operating Room Department is staffed with 2 nursing supervisors on the day shift and 1 nursing supervisor apiece on the evening and night shifts. There are 2 technicians on the day shift, 2 technicians on the evening shift, and 1 technician on the night shift. There are 3 RNs on the day shift, 2 RNs on the evening shift, and 1 RN plus 1 LPN on the night shift. In addition there is one aide plus one clerical on the day shift only.

Required

1. Set up a staffing requirements worksheet, using the format in Exhibit 8–4.
2. Compute the number of FTEs required to fill the Operating Room staffing positions.

CHAPTER 9

Example 9A: Common Sizing

Common sizing converts numbers to percentages so that comparative analysis can be performed. Reread the chapter text about common sizing and examine the percentages shown in Table 9–1.

Practice Exercise 9–I: Common Sizing

The worksheet below shows the assets of two hospitals.

Required

Perform common sizing for the assets of the two hospitals.

	Same Year for Both Hospitals	
	Hospital A	Hospital B
Current Assets	$ 2,000,000	$ 8,000,000
Property, Plant & Equipment	7,500,000	30,000,000
Other Assets	500,000	2,000,000
Total Assets	$10,000,000	$40,000,000

Assignment Exercise 9–1: Common Sizing

Refer to the Metropolis Health System (MHS) comparative financial statements at the back of the Examples and Exercises section.

Required

Common size the MHS Statement of Revenue and Expenses.

Example 9B: Trend Analysis

Trend analysis allows comparison of figures over time. Reread the chapter text about trend analysis and examine the *difference* columns shown in Table 9–3.

Practice Exercise 9–II: Trend Analysis

The worksheet below shows the assets of Hospital A over two years.

Required

Perform trend analysis for the assets of Hospital A.

	Hospital A	
	Year 1	Year 2
Current Assets	$1,600,000	$ 2,000,000
Property, Plant & Equipment	6,000,000	7,500,000
Other Assets	400,000	500,000
Total Assets	$8,000,000	$10,000,000

Assignment Exercise 9–2: Trend Analysis

Refer to the Metropolis Health System (MHS) comparative financial statements at the back of the Examples and Exercises section.

Required

Perform trend analysis on the MHS Statement of Revenue and Expenses.

CHAPTER 10

Example 10A: Budgeting

A static budget is based on a single level of operations, which is never adjusted. Therefore the static budgeted expense amounts will not change even though actual volume does change during the year.

The computation of a static budget variance only requires one calculation, as follows:

Actual		*Static budget*		*Static budget*
results	minus	*amount*	equals	*variance*

We can set up the example in the chapter text in this format as follows.

Use patient days as an example of level of volume, or output. Assume that the budget anticipated 40,000 patient days this year at an average of $600 revenue per day, or $24,000,000. Further assume that expenses were budgeted at $560 per patient day, or $22,400,000. The budget would look like this:

	As Budgeted
Revenue	$24,000,000
Expenses	22,400,000
Excess of Revenue over Expenses	$ 1,600,000

Now assume that only 36,000, or 90 percent, of the patient days are going to actually be achieved for the year. The average revenue of $600 per day will be achieved for these 36,000 days (thus 36,000 times 600 equals 21,600,000). Further assume that, despite the best efforts of the Chief Financial Officer, the expenses will amount to $22,000,000. The actual results would look like this:

	Actual
Revenue	$21,600,000
Expenses	22,000,000
Excess of Expenses over Revenue	$ (400,000)

The budgeted revenue and expenses still reflect the original expectation of 40,000 patient days; the budget report would look like this:

	Actual	Budget	Static Budget Variance
Revenue	$21,600,000	$24,000,000	$(2,400,000)
Expenses	22,000,000	22,400,000	(400,000)
Excess of Expenses over Revenue	$ (400,000)	$ 1,600,000	$(2,000,000)

Note: The negative actual result of (400,000) combined with the positive budget expectation of 1,600,000 amounts to the negative net variance of (2,000,000).

This example has shown a static budget, geared toward only one level of activity and remaining constant or static.

Practice Exercise 10–I: Budgeting

Budget assumptions for this exercise include both inpatient and outpatient revenue and expense. Assumptions are as follows:

As to the initial budget:

The budget anticipated 30,000 inpatient days this year at an average of $650 revenue per day.

- Inpatient expenses were budgeted at $600 per patient day.
- The budget anticipated 10,000 outpatient visits this year at an average of $400 revenue per visit.
- Outpatient expenses were budgeted at $380 per visit.

As to the actual results:

- Assume that only 27,000, or 90 percent, of the inpatient days are going to actually be achieved for the year.
- The average revenue of $650 per day will be achieved for these 27,000 inpatient days.
- The outpatient visits will actually amount to 110 percent, or 11,000 for the year.
- The average revenue of $400 per visit will be achieved for these 11,000 visits.
- Further assume that, due to the heroic efforts of the Chief Financial Officer, the actual inpatient expenses will amount to $11,600,000 and the actual outpatient expenses will amount to $4,000,000.

Required

1. Set up three worksheets that follow the format of those in Example 10A. However, in each of your worksheets make two lines for Revenue; label one as *Revenue-Inpatient* and the other *Revenue-Outpatient*. Add a *Revenue Subtotal* line. Likewise, make two lines for *Expense*; label one as *Expense-Inpatient* and the other *Expense-Outpatient*. Add an *Expense Subtotal* line.

2. Using the new assumptions, complete the first worksheet for "As Budgeted."
3. Using the new assumptions, complete the second worksheet for "Actual."
4. Using the new assumptions, complete the third worksheet for "Static Budget Variance."

Assignment Exercise 10–1: Budgeting

Select an organization; either Metropolis Health System from the Chapter 15 Case Study or one of the organizations presented in the three Mini-Case Studies in Chapter 16.

Required

1. Using the organization selected, create a budget for the next fiscal year. Set out the details of all assumptions you needed in order to build this budget.
2. Use the Checklist for Building a Budget (Exhibit 10–2) and critique your own budget.

Assignment Exercise 10–2: Budgeting

Find an existing budget from a published source. Detail should be extensive enough to present a challenge.

Required

1. Using the existing budget, create a new budget for the next fiscal year. Set out the details of all assumptions you needed in order to build this budget.
2. Use the Checklist for Building a Budget (Exhibit 10–2) and critique your own effort.
3. Use the Checklist for Reviewing a Budget (Exhibit 10–1) and critique the existing budget.

Example 10B: Variance Analysis

Our variance analysis example and practice exercise use the flexible budget approach. A flexible budget is one that is created using budgeted revenue and/or budgeted cost amounts. A flexible budget is adjusted, or flexed, to the actual level of output achieved (or perhaps expected to be achieved) during the budget period. A flexible budget thus looks toward a range of activity or volume (versus only one level in the static budget).

Examples of how the variance analysis works are contained in Figure 10–1 (the elements), in Figure 10–2 (the composition), and in Figures 10–3 and 10–4 (the calculation). Study these examples before undertaking the Practice Exercise.

Practice Exercise 10–II: Variance Analysis

Exhibit 10–4 presents a Summary Variance Report for the nursing activity center of St. Joseph Hospital for the month of September. For our practice exercise we will duplicate this report for the month of March.

Assumptions are as follows:

- Actual Activity Level is 687,000.
- Budgeted Activity Level is 650,000.

- Actual Cost per RVU is $4.70.
- Budgeted Cost per RVU is $5.00.
- Actual Overhead Costs are $3,228,900.
- Budgeted Overhead Costs are $3,250,000.

Required

1. Set up a worksheet for the month of March like that shown in Exhibit 10–4 for the month of September.
2. Insert the March Input Data (per assumptions given above) on the worksheet.
3. Complete the "Actual Costs," "Flexible Budget," and "Budgeted Costs" sections at the top of the worksheet.
4. Compute the Price Variance and the Quantity Variance in the middle of the worksheet.
5. Indicate whether the Price and the Quantity Variances are favorable or unfavorable for March.

Optional

Can you compute how the $3,228,900 actual overhead costs and the $3,250,000 budgeted overhead costs were calculated?

Assignment Exercise 10–3: Variance Analysis

Greenview Hospital operated at 120 percent of normal capacity in two of its departments during the year. It operated 120 percent times 20,000 normal capacity direct labor nursing hours in routine services and it operated 120 percent times 20,000 normal capacity equipment hours in the laboratory. The lab allocates overhead by measuring minutes and hours the equipment is used; thus *equipment hours*.

Assumptions:

For Routine Services Nursing:

- 20,000 hours × 120% = 24,000 direct labor nursing hours.
- Budgeted Overhead at 24,000 hours = $42,000 fixed plus $6,000 variable = $48,000 total.
- Actual Overhead at 24,000 hours = $42,000 fixed plus $7,000 variable = $49,000 total.
- Applied Overhead for 24,000 hours at $2.35 @ = $56,400.

For Laboratory:

- 20,000 hours × 120% = 24,000 equipment hours.
- Budgeted Overhead at 24,000 hours = $59,600 fixed plus $11,400 variable = $71,000 total.
- Actual Overhead at 24,000 hours = $59,600 fixed plus $11,600 variable = $71,200 total.
- Applied Overhead for 24,000 hours at $3.455 @ = $82,920.

Required

1. Set up a worksheet for Applied Overhead Costs and Volume Variance with a column for Routine Services Nursing and a second column for Laboratory.

2. Set up a worksheet for Actual Overhead Costs and Budget Variance with a column for Routine Services Nursing and a second column for Laboratory.
3. Set up a worksheet for Volume Variance and Budget Variance totaling Net Variance with a column for Routine Services Nursing and a second column for Laboratory.
4. Insert input data from Assumptions.
5. Complete computations for all three worksheets

CHAPTER 11

Example 11A: Unadjusted Rate of Return

Assumptions:

- Average annual net income = $100,000
- Original investment amount = $1,000,000
- Unrecovered asset cost at the end of useful life (salvage value) = $100,000

Calculation using original investment amount:

$$\frac{\$100,000}{\$1,000,000} = 10\% \text{ Unadjusted Rate of Return}$$

Calculation using average investment amount:

First Step: Compute average investment amount for total unrecovered asset cost.

At beginning of estimated useful life	=	$1,000,000
At end of estimated useful life	=	$ 100,000
	Sum	$1,100,000

Divided by 2 = $550,000 average investment amount

Second Step: Calculate unadjusted rate of return.

$$\frac{\$100,000}{\$550,000} = 18.2\% \text{ Unadjusted Rate of Return}$$

Practice Exercise 11–I: Unadjusted Rate of Return

Assumptions:

- Average annual net income = $100,000
- Original investment amount = $500,000
- Unrecovered asset cost at the end of useful life (salvage value) = $50,000

Required

1. Compute the Unadjusted Rate of Return using the original investment amount.
2. Compute the Unadjusted Rate of Return using the average investment method.

Assignment Exercise 11–1: Unadjusted Rate of Return

Metropolis Health Systems' Laboratory Director expects to purchase a new piece of equipment. The assumptions for the transaction are as follows:

- Average annual net income = $70,000
- Original investment amount = $410,000
- Unrecovered asset cost at the end of useful life (salvage value) = $41,000

Required

1. Compute the Unadjusted Rate of Return using the original investment amount.
2. Compute the Unadjusted Rate of Return using the average investment method.

Example 11B: Finding the Future Value (with a Compound Interest Table)

Betty Dylan is Director of Nurses at Metropolis Health System. Her oldest son will be entering college in five years. Today Betty is trying to figure what his college fund will amount to in five more years. (Hint: Compound interest means interest is not only earned on the principal, but also is earned on the previous interest earnings that have been left in the account. Interest is thus *compounded*.)

The college fund savings account presently has a balance of $9,000 and any interest earned over the next five years will be left in the account. Betty assumes the annual interest rate will be 6 percent. How much money will be in the account at the end of five more years?

Solution to Example

Step 1. Refer to the Compound Interest Table found in Appendix 11B at the back of this chapter. Reading across, or horizontally, find the 6 percent column. Reading down, or vertically, find Year 5. Trace across the Year 5 line item to the 6 percent column. The factor is 1.338.

Step 2. Multiply the current savings account balance of $9,000 times the factor of 1.338 to find the future value of $12,042. In five years at compound interest of 6 percent the college fund will have a balance of $12,042.

Practice Exercise 11–II: Finding the Future Value (with a Compound Interest Table)

Assume the college savings fund in the preceding example presently has a balance of $11,000 and any interest earned will be left in the account. Assume the annual interest rate will be 7 percent.

Required

Compute how much money will be in the account at the end of six more years. (Use the Future Value or Compound Interest Table found at the back of this chapter.)

Assignment Exercise 11–2: Finding the Future Value (with a Compound Interest Table)

John Whitten is one of the physicians on staff at Metropolis Health System. His practice is six years old. He has set up an office savings account to accumulate the funds to replace equipment in his practice. Today John is trying to figure what his equipment fund will amount to in four more years.

The equipment fund savings account presently has a balance of $63,500 and any interest earned over the next four years will be left in the account. John assumes the annual interest rate will be 5 percent. How much money will be in the account at the end of four more years?

Required

Compute how much money will be in the account at the end of four more years. (Use the Future Value or Compound Interest Table found at the back of this chapter.)

Example 11C: Finding the Present Value (with a Present Value Table)

Betty Dylan is taking an adult education night course in personal finance at the community college. The class is presently studying retirement planning. Each student is to estimate the amount of funds (in addition to pension plans and social security) they believe will be needed at retirement. Then they are to make a retirement plan.

Betty has estimated she would need $100,000 fifteen years from now. In order to complete her assignment she needs to know the present value of the $100,000. Betty further assumes an interest rate of 6 percent.

Solution to Example

Step 1. Refer to the Present Value Table found in Appendix 11-A at the back of this chapter. Reading across, or horizontally, find the 6 percent column. Reading down, or vertically, find Year 15. Trace across the Year 15 line item to the 6 percent column. The factor is 0.4173.

Step 2. Multiply $100,000 times the factor of 0.4173 to find the present value of $41,730.

Practice Exercise 11–III: Finding the Present Value (with a Present Value Table)

Betty isn't finished with her assignment. Now she wants to find the present value of $150,000 accumulated fifteen years from now. She further assumes a better interest rate of 7 percent.

Required

Compute the present value of $150,000 accumulated fifteen years from now. Assume an interest rate of 7 percent. (Use the Present Value Table found at the back of this chapter.)

Assignment Exercise 11–3: Finding the Present Value (with a Present Value Table)

Part 1—Dr. John Whitten is still figuring on his equipment fund. According to his calculations he needs $250,000 to be accumulated six years from now. John is now trying to find the present value of the $250,000. He continues to assume an interest rate of 5 percent.

Required

Compute the present value of $250,000 accumulated fifteen years from now. Assume an interest rate of 5 percent. (Use the Present Value Table found at the back of this chapter.)

Part 2—John doesn't like the answer he gets. What, he thinks, if he can raise the interest rate to 7 percent? How much difference would that make?

Required

Compute the present value of $250,000 accumulated fifteen years from now assuming an interest rate of 7 percent. Compare the difference between this amount and the present value at 5 percent.

Example 11D: Internal Rate of Return

Review the chapter text to follow the steps set out to compute internal rate of return.

Practice Exercise 11–IV: Internal Rate of Return

Metropolis Health System (MHS) is considering purchasing a tractor to mow the grounds. It would cost $16,950 and have a 10-year useful life. It will have zero salvage value at the end of 10 years. The head of the MHS grounds crew estimates it would save $3,000 per year. He figures this savings because just one of the present maintenance crew would be driving the tractor, replacing the labor of several men now using small household-type lawn mowers. Compute the internal rate of return for this proposed acquisition.

Assignment Exercise 11–4: Computing an Internal Rate of Return

Dr. Whitten has decided to purchase equipment that has a cost of $60,000 and will produce a pretax net cash inflow of $30,000 per year over its estimated useful life of six years. The equipment will have no salvage value and will be depreciated by the straight-line method. The tax rate is 50 percent. Determine Dr. Whitten's approximate after-tax internal rate of return.

Example 11E: Payback Period

Review the chapter text and follow the Doctor Green detailed example of payback period computation.

Practice Exercise 11–V: Payback

The MHS Chief Financial Officer is considering a request by the Emergency Room Department for purchase of new equipment. It will cost $500,000. There is no trade-in. Its useful life would be 10 years. This type of machine is new to the department but it is estimated that it will result in $84,000 annual revenue and operating costs would be one-quarter of that amount. The CFO wants to find the payback period for this piece of equipment.

Assignment Exercise 11–5: Payback Period

The MHS Chief Financial Officer is considering alternate proposals for the hospital radiology department. The Director of Radiology has suggested purchasing one of two pieces of equipment. Machine A costs $15,000 and Machine B costs $12,000. Both machines are estimated to reduce radiology operating costs by $5,000 per year.

Required

Which machine should be purchased? Make your payback calculations to provide the answer. Assume the useful life is 10 years.

CHAPTER 12

Practice Exercise 12–I: Components of Balance Sheet and Statement of Net Income

Financial Statements for Doctors Smith and Brown are provided below. Use the doctors' Balance Sheet, Statement of Revenue and Expenses, and Statement of Capital for this assignment.

Required

Identify the following doctors' Balance Sheet and Statement of Net Income components. List the name of each component and its amount(s) from the appropriate financial statement.

> Current Liabilities
> Total Assets
> Income from Operations
> Accumulated Depreciation
> Total Operating Revenue
> Current Portion of Long-Term Debt
> Interest Income
> Inventories

Assignment Exercise 12–1: Components of Balance Sheet and Statement of Net Income

Refer to the Metropolis Health System (MHS) Supplemental Information at the back of the Examples and Exercises section. Use the MHS comparative Balance Sheet, Statement of Revenue and Expenses, and Statement of Fund Balance for this assignment.

Required

Identify the following MHS Balance Sheet components. List the name of each component and its amount(s) from the appropriate MHS financial statement.

> Current Liabilities
> Total Assets
> Income from Operations
> Accumulated Depreciation
> Total Operating Revenue
> Current Portion of Long-Term Debt
> Interest Income

Doctors Smith and Brown
Statement of Net Income
for the Three Months Ended March 31, 2000

Revenue		
Net patient service revenue	180,000	
Other revenue	-0-	
Total Operating Revenue		180,000
Expenses		
Nursing/PA salaries	16,650	
Clerical salaries	10,150	
Payroll taxes/employee benefits	4,800	
Medical supplies and drugs	15,000	
Professional fees	3,000	
Dues and publications	2,400	
Janitorial service	1,200	
Office supplies	1,500	
Repairs and maintenance	1,200	
Utilities and telephone	6,000	
Depreciation	30,000	
Interest	3,100	
Other	5,000	
Total Expenses		100,000
Income from Operations		80,000
Nonoperating Gains (Losses)		
Interest Income		-0-
Nonoperating Gains, Net		-0-
Net Income		80,000

Doctors Smith and Brown
Balance Sheet
March 31, 2000

Assets

Current Assets		
Cash and cash equivalents	25,000	
Patient accounts receivable	40,000	
Inventories—supplies and drugs	5,000	
Total Current Assets		70,000
Property, Plant and Equipment		
Buildings and Improvements	500,000	
Equipment	800,000	
Total	1,300,000	
Less Accumulated Depreciation	(480,000)	
Net Depreciable Assets	820,000	
Land	100,000	
Property, Plant and Equipment, Net		920,000
Other Assets		10,000
Total Assets		1,000,000

Liabilities and Capital

Current Liabilities		
Current maturities of long-term debt	10,000	
Accounts payable and accrued expenses	20,000	
Total Current Liabilities		30,000
Long-Term Debt	180,000	
Less Current Portion of Long-Term Debt	(10,000)	
Net Long-Term Debt		170,000
Total Liabilities		200,000
Capital		800,000
Total Liabilities and Capital		1,000,000

Doctors Smith and Brown
Statement of Changes in Capital
for the Three Months Ended March 31, 2000

Beginning Balance	$720,000
Net Income	80,000
Ending Balance	$800,000

Example 12B: Depreciation Concept

Assume that MHS purchased equipment for $200,000 cash on April 1st (the first day of its fiscal year). This equipment has an expected life of 10 years. The salvage value is 10 percent of cost. No equipment was traded in on this purchase.

Straight-line depreciation is a method that charges an equal amount of depreciation for each year the asset is in service. In the case of this purchase, straight-line depreciation would amount to $18,000 per year for 10 years. This amount is computed as follows:

Step 1. Compute the cost net of salvage or trade-in value: 200,000 less 10 percent salvage value or 20,000 equals 180,000.

Step 2. Divide the resulting figure by the expected life (also known as estimated useful life): 180,000 divided by 10 equals 18,000 depreciation per year for 10 years.

Accelerated depreciation represents methods that are speeded up, or accelerated. In other words a greater amount of depreciation is taken earlier in the life of the asset. One example of accelerated depreciation is the double declining balance method. Unlike straight-line depreciation, trade-in or salvage value is not taken into account until the end of the depreciation schedule. This method uses *book value*, which is the net amount remaining when cumulative previous depreciation is deducted from the asset's cost. The computation is as follows:

Step 1. Compute the straight-line rate: 1 divided by 10 equals 10 percent.

Step 2. Now double the rate (as in *double declining method*): 10 percent times 2 equals 20 percent.

Step 3. Compute the first year's depreciation expense: 200,000 times 20 percent equals 40,000.

Step 4. Compute the carry-forward book value at the beginning of the second year: 200,000 book value beginning Year 1 less Year 1 depreciation of 40,000 equals book value at beginning of the second year of 160,000.

Step 5. Compute the second year's depreciation expense: 160,000 times 20 percent equals 32,000.

Step 6. Compute the carry-forward book value at the beginning of the third year:
160,000 book value beginning Year 2 less Year 2 depreciation of 32,000 equals book value at beginning of the third year of 128,000.
—Continue until the asset's salvage or trade-in value has been reached.
—Do not depreciate beyond the salvage or trade-in value.

Practice Exercise 12–II: Depreciation Concept

Assume that MHS purchased equipment for $600,000 cash on April 1st (the first day of its fiscal year). This equipment has an expected life of 10 years. The salvage value is 10 percent of cost. No equipment was traded in on this purchase.

Required

1. Compute the straight-line depreciation for this purchase.
2. Compute the double declining balance depreciation for this purchase.

Assignment Exercise 12–2: Depreciation Concept

Assume that MHS purchased two additional pieces of equipment on April 1st (the first day of its fiscal year), as follows:

(1) The laboratory equipment cost $300,000 and has an expected life of 5 years. The salvage value is 5 percent of cost. No equipment was traded in on this purchase.

(2) The radiology equipment cost $800,000 and has an expected life of 7 years. The salvage value is 10 percent of cost. No equipment was traded in on this purchase.

Required

For both pieces of equipment:
1. Compute the straight-line depreciation.
2. Compute the double declining balance depreciation.

CHAPTER 13

Example 13A

To better understand how the information for the numerator and the denominator of each calculation is obtained, Figure 13–1, Examples of Liquidity Ratio Calculations, illustrates the process. This figure takes the balance sheet and the statement of revenue and expense that were discussed in the preceding chapter and illustrates the source of each figure in the four liquidity ratios. The multiple computations in Days Cash on Hand and in Days Receivables are further broken out into a three-step process to better illustrate sources of information.

Practice Exercise 13–I: Liquidity Ratios

Two of the liquidity ratios are illustrated in this practice exercise. Refer to the Doctors Smith and Brown financial statements presented in preceding Chapter 12.

Required

1. Set up a worksheet for the current ratio and the quick ratio.
2. Compute the ratios for Doctors Smith and Brown.

Assignment Exercise 13–1: Liquidity Ratios

Refer to the Metropolis Health System (MHS) case study in Chapter 15.

Required

1. Set up a worksheet for the liquidity ratios.
2. Compute the four liquidity ratios using the Chapter 15 MHS financial statements.

Example 13B

To better understand how the information for the numerator and the denominator of each calculation is obtained, Figure 13–2, Examples of Solvency and Profitability Ratio Calculations, illustrates the process. This figure takes the balance sheet and the statement of revenue and expense that were discussed in the preceding chapter and illustrates the source of each figure in the two solvency ratios. Any multiple computations are further broken out to better explain sources of information.

Practice Exercise 13–II: Solvency Ratios

Refer to the Doctors Smith and Brown financial statements presented in preceding Chapter 12.

Required

1. Set up a worksheet for the solvency ratios.
2. Compute these ratios for Doctors Smith and Brown. To do so, you will need one additional piece of information that is not present on the doctors' statements: their maximum annual debt service is $22,200.

Assignment Exercise 13–2: Solvency Ratios

Refer to the Metropolis Health System (MHS) case study in Chapter 15.

Required

1. Set up a worksheet for the liquidity ratios.
2. Compute the solvency ratios using the Chapter 15 MHS financial statements.

Example 13C

To better understand how the information for the numerator and the denominator of each calculation is obtained, study Figure 13–2, Examples of Solvency and Profitability Ratio Calculations. This figure takes the balance sheet and the statement of revenue and expense that were discussed in the preceding chapter and illustrates the source of each figure in the two profitability ratios. Any multiple computations are further broken out to better explain sources of information.

Practice Exercise 13–III: Profitability Ratios

Refer to the Doctors Smith and Brown financial statements presented in preceding Chapter 12.

Required

1. Set up a worksheet for the profitability ratios.
2. Compute these ratios for Doctors Smith and Brown. All the necessary information is present on the doctors' statements.
   [Hint: "Operating Income (Loss)" is also known as "Income from Operations."]

Assignment Exercise 13–3: Profitability Ratios

Refer to the Metropolis Health System (MHS) case study in Chapter 15.

Required

1. Set up a worksheet for the liquidity ratios.
2. Compute the profitability ratios using the Chapter 15 MHS financial statements.

CHAPTER 14

Assignment Exercise 14–1: Quartiles

Review the chapter text about quartiles and study Table 14–1, which indicates results in quartiles.

Required

1. Refer to Exhibit 14–1. Use the 12-month totals in Exhibit 14–1 to divide the District 8 hospitals into quartiles.
2. Enter your results on a worksheet with the highest quartile first and the lowest quartile last.

Assignment Exercise 14–2: Benchmarking

Review the chapter text about benchmarking. Examine Table 14–1, which is an example of thirteen different benchmarking measures.

Required

1. Select either the MHS case study in Chapter 15 or one of the organizations represented by a mini-case study in Chapter 16.
2. Prepare a list of measures that could be benchmarked for this organization. Comment on why these items are important for benchmarking purposes.
3. Find another example of benchmarking for a health care organization. The example can be an organization report or it can be taken from a published source such as a journal article.

Assignment Exercise 14–3: Pareto Rule

Review the chapter text about the Pareto rule and examine Figure 14–2. Note that the text says Pareto diagrams are often drawn to reflect *before* and *after* results.

Assume that Figure 14–2 is the *before* diagram for the Billing Department. Further assume that the *after* results are as follows:

Activity	Activity Code	Number
Process Denied Bills	PDB	12
Review with Supervisor	RWS	10
Locate Documentation	LD	6
Copy Documentation	CD	5
		33

Required

1. Redo the Pareto diagram with the *after* results. (Use Figure 14–2 as a guide.)
2. Comment on the *before* and *after* results for the Billing Department.

SUPPLEMENTAL MATERIALS

Present Value of an Annuity of $1

Periods	2%	4%	6%	8%	10%	12%	14%	16%	18%	20%	Periods
1	.980	.962	.943	.926	.909	.893	.877	.862	.848	.833	1
2	1.942	1.886	1.833	1.783	1.736	1.690	1.647	1.605	1.566	1.528	2
3	2.884	2.775	2.673	2.577	2.487	2.402	2.322	2.246	2.174	2.107	3
4	3.808	3.630	3.465	3.312	3.170	3.037	2.914	2.798	2.690	2.589	4
5	4.713	4.452	4.212	3.993	3.791	3.605	3.433	3.274	3.127	2.991	5
6	5.601	5.242	4.917	4.623	4.355	4.111	3.889	3.685	3.498	3.326	6
7	6.472	6.002	5.582	5.206	4.868	4.564	4.288	4.039	3.812	3.605	7
8	7.325	6.733	6.210	5.747	5.335	4.968	4.639	4.344	4.078	3.837	8
9	8.162	7.435	6.802	6.247	5.759	5.328	4.946	4.607	4.303	4.031	9
10	8.983	8.111	7.360	6.710	6.145	5.650	5.216	4.833	4.494	4.193	10
15	12.849	11.118	9.712	8.560	7.606	6.811	6.142	5.576	5.092	4.676	15
20	16.351	13.590	11.470	9.818	8.514	7.469	6.623	5.929	5.353	4.870	20
25	19.523	15.622	12.783	10.675	9.077	7.843	6.873	6.097	5.467	4.948	25

Metropolis Health System
Balance Sheet
March 31, 2000, and 1999

Assets

Current Assets		
Cash and cash equivalents	1,150,000	400,000
Assets whose use is limited	825,000	825,000
Patient accounts receivable	8,700,000	8,950,000
Less allowance for bad debts	(1,300,000)	(1,300,000)
Other receivables	150,000	100,000
Inventories of supplies	900,000	850,000
Prepaid expenses	200,000	150,000
Total Current Assets	10,625,000	9,975,000
Assets Whose Use is Limited		
Corporate funded depreciation	1,950,000	1,800,000
Under bond indenture agreements—		
held by trustee	1,425,000	1,475,000
Total Assets Whose Use is Limited	3,375,000	3,275,000
Less Current Portion	(825,000)	(825,000)
Net Assets Whose Use is Limited	2,550,000	2,450,000
Property, Plant and Equipment, Net	19,300,000	19,200,000
Other Assets	325,000	375,000
Total Assets	32,800,000	32,000,000

Metropolis Health System
Balance Sheet
March 31, 2000, and 1999

Liabilities and Fund Balance

Current Liabilities		
Current maturities of long-term debt	525,000	500,000
Accounts payable and accrued expenses	4,900,000	5,300,000
Bond interest payable	300,000	325,000
Reimbursement settlement payable	100,000	175,000
Total Current Liabilities	5,825,000	6,300,000
Long-Term Debt	6,000,000	6,500,000
Less Current Portion of Long-Term Debt	(525,000)	(500,000)
Net Long-Term Debt	5,475,000	6,000,000
Total Liabilities	11,300,000	12,300,000
Fund Balances		
General Fund	21,500,000	19,700,000
Total Fund Balances	21,500,000	19,700,000
Total Liabilities and Fund Balances	32,800,000	32,000,000

Metropolis Health System
Statement of Revenue and Expenses
for the Years Ended March 31, 2000, and 1999

Revenue
Net patient service revenue	34,000,000		33,600,000	
Other revenue	1,100,000		1,000,000	
Total Operating Revenue		35,100,000		34,600,000

Expenses
Nursing services	5,025,000		5,450,000	
Other professional services	13,100,000		12,950,000	
General services	3,200,000		3,220,000	
Support services	8,300,000		8,340,000	
Depreciation	1,900,000		1,800,000	
Amortization	50,000		50,000	
Interest	325,000		350,000	
Provision for doubtful accounts	1,500,000		1,600,000	
Total Expenses		33,400,000		33,760,000
Income from Operations		1,700,000		840,000

Nonoperating Gains (Losses)
Unrestricted gifts and memorials	20,000		70,000	
Interest income	80,000		40,000	
Nonoperating Gains, Net		100,000		110,000

Revenue and Gains in Excess of Expenses and Losses		1,800,000		950,000

Metropolis Health System
Statement of Changes in Fund Balance
for the Years Ended March 31, 2000, and 1999

General Fund Balance April 1st	$19,700,000	$18,750,000
Revenue and Gains in Excess of Expenses and Losses	1,800,000	950,000
General Fund Balance March 31st	$21,500,000	$19,700,000

Metropolis Health System
Schedule of Property, Plant, and Equipment
for the Years Ended March 31, 2000, and 1999

Buildings and Improvements	14,700,000	14,000,000
Land Improvements	1,100,000	1,100,000
Equipment	28,900,000	27,600,000
Total	44,700,000	42,700,000
Less Accumulated Depreciation	(26,100,000)	(24,200,000)
Net Depreciable Assets	18,600,000	18,500,000
Land	480,000	480,000
Construction in Progress	220,000	220,000
Net Property, Plant, and Equipment	19,300,000	19,200,000

Metropolis Health System
Schedule of Patient Revenue
for the Years Ended March 31, 2000, and 1999

Patient Services Revenue

Routine revenue	9,850,000	9,750,000
Laboratory	7,375,000	7,300,000
Radiology and CT scanner	5,825,000	5,760,000
OB–nursery	450,000	445,000
Pharmacy	3,175,000	3,140,000
Emergency service	2,200,000	2,180,000
Medical and surgical supply and IV	5,050,000	5,000,000
Operating rooms	5,250,000	5,200,000
Anesthesiology	1,600,000	1,580,000
Respiratory therapy	900,000	890,000
Physical therapy	1,475,000	1,460,000
EKG and EEG	1,050,000	1,040,000
Ambulance services	900,000	890,000
Oxygen	575,000	570,000
Home health and hospice	1,675,000	1,660,000
Substance abuse	375,000	370,000
Other	775,000	765,000
Subtotal	48,500,000	48,000,000
Less: Allowances and Charity Care	14,500,000	14,400,000
Net Patient Service Revenue	34,000,000	33,600,000

Metropolis Health System
Schedule of Operating Expenses
for the Years Ended March 31, 2000, and 1999

Nursing Services		
Routine Medical-Surgical	3,880,000	4,200,000
Operating Room	300,000	325,000
Intensive Care Units	395,000	430,000
OB–Nursery	150,000	165,000
Other	300,000	330,000
Total	5,025,000	5,450,000
Other Professional Services		
Laboratory	2,375,000	2,350,000
Radiology and CT Scanner	1,700,000	1,680,000
Pharmacy	1,375,000	1,360,000
Emergency Service	950,000	930,000
Medical and Surgical Supply	1,800,000	1,780,000
Operating Rooms and Anesthesia	1,525,000	1,515,000
Respiratory Therapy	525,000	530,000
Physical Therapy	700,000	695,000
EKG and EEG	185,000	180,000
Ambulance Services	80,000	80,000
Substance Abuse	460,000	450,000
Home Health and Hospice	1,295,000	1,280,000
Other	130,000	120,000
Total	13,100,000	12,950,000
General Services		
Dietary	1,055,000	1,060,000
Maintenance	1,000,000	1,010,000
Laundry	295,000	300,000
Housekeeping	470,000	475,000
Security	50,000	50,000
Medical Records	330,000	325,000
Total	3,200,000	3,220,000
Support Services		
General	4,600,000	4,540,000
Insurance	240,000	235,000
Payroll Taxes	1,130,000	1,180,000
Employee Welfare	1,900,000	1,950,000
Other	430,000	435,000
Total	8,300,000	8,340,000

continues

Metropolis Health System
Schedule of Operating Expenses
for the Years Ended March 31, 2000, and 1999
continued

Depreciation	1,900,000	1,800,000
Amortization	50,000	50,000
Interest Expense	325,000	350,000
Provision for Doubtful Accounts	1,500,000	1,600,000
Total Operating Expenses	33,400,000	33,760,000

EXCERPTS FROM METROPOLITAN HEALTH SYSTEM NOTES TO FINANCIAL STATEMENTS

Note 1—Nature of Operations and Summary of Significant Accounting Policies

General

Metropolitan Hospital System (Hospital) currently operates as a general acute care hospital. The Hospital is a municipal corporation and body politic created under the Hospital District laws of the State.

Cash and Cash Equivalents

For purposes of reporting cash flows, the Hospital considers all liquid investments with an original maturity of three months or less to be cash equivalents.

Inventory

Inventory consists of supplies used for patients and is stated at the lower of cost or market. Cost is determined on the basis of most recent purchase price.

Investments

Investments, consisting primarily of debt securities, are carried at market value. Realized and unrealized gains and losses are reflected in the statement of revenue and expenses. Investment income from general fund investments is reported as nonoperating gains.

Income Taxes

As a municipal corporation of the State, the Hospital is exempt from Federal and State income taxes under Section 115 of the Internal Revenue Code.

Property, Plant, and Equipment

Expenditures for property, plant, and equipment and items that substantially increase the useful lives of existing assets are capitalized at cost. The Hospital provides for depreciation on the straight-line method at rates designed to depreciate the costs of assets over estimated useful lives as follows:

	Years
Equipment	5 to 20
Land Improvements	20 to 25
Buildings and Improvements	40

Funded Depreciation

The Hospital's Board of Directors has adopted the policy of designating certain funds that are to be used to fund depreciation for the purpose of improvement, replacement, or expansion of plant assets.

Unamortized Debt Issue Costs

Revenue bond issue costs have been deferred and are being amortized.

Revenue and Gains in Excess of Expenses and Losses

The statement of revenue and expenses includes Revenue and Gains in Excess of Expenses and Losses. Changes in unrestricted net assets that are excluded from excess of revenue over expenses, consistent with industry practice, would include such items as contributions of long-lived assets (including assets acquired using contributions that by donor restriction were to be used for the purposes of acquiring such assets) and extraordinary gains and losses. Such items are not present on the current financial statements.

Net Patient Service Revenue

Net patient service revenue is reported at the estimated net realizable amounts from patients, third-party payers, and others for services rendered, including estimated retroactive adjustments under reimbursement agreements with third-party payers. Retroactive adjustments are accrued on an estimated basis in the period the related services are rendered and adjusted in future periods as final settlements are determined.

Contractual Agreements with Third-Party Payers

The Hospital has contractual agreements with third-party payers, primarily the Medicare and Medicaid programs. The Medicare program reimburses the Hospital for inpatient services under the Prospective Payment System, which provides for payment at predetermined amounts based on the discharge diagnosis. The contractual agreement with the Medicaid program provides for reimbursement based upon rates established by the State, subject to State appropriations. The difference between established customary charge rates and reimbursement is accounted for as a contractual allowance.

Gifts and Bequests

Unrestricted gifts and bequests are recorded on the accrual basis as nonoperating gains.

Donated Services

No amounts have been reflected in the financial statements for donated services. The Hospital pays for most services requiring specific expertise. However, many individuals volunteer their time and perform a variety of tasks that assists the Hospital with specific assistance programs and various committee assignments.

NOTE 2—CASH AND INVESTMENTS

Statutes require that all deposits of the Hospital be secured by federal depository insurance or be fully collateralized by the banking institution in authorized investments. Authorized investments include those guaranteed by the full faith and credit of the United States of America as to principal and interest; or in bonds, notes, debentures, or other similar obligations of the United States of America or its agencies; in interest-bearing savings accounts, interest-bearing certificates of deposit; or in certain money market mutual funds.

At March 31, 2000, the carrying amount and bank balance of the Hospital's deposits with financial institutions were $190,000 and $227,000, respectively. The difference between the carrying amount and the bank balance primarily represents checks outstanding at March 31, 2000. All deposits are fully insured by the Federal Deposit Insurance Corporation or collateralized with securities held in the Hospital's name by the Hospital agent.

	Carrying Amount	
	2000	*1999*
U.S. Government Securities or		
U.S. Government Agency Securities	4,325,000	3,575,000
Total Investments	4,325,000	3,575,000
Petty Cash	3,000	3,000
Deposits	190,000	93,000
Accrued Interest	7,000	4,000
Total	4,525,000	3,675,000
Consisting of		
Cash and Cash Equivalents—General Fund	1,150,000	400,000
Assets Whose Use Is Limited		
Corporate Funded Depreciation	1,950,000	1,800,000
Held by Trustee under Bond Indenture Agreements	1,425,000	1,475,000
Total	4,525,000	3,675,000

NOTE 3—CHARITY CARE

The Hospital voluntarily provides free care to patients who lack financial resources and are deemed to be medically indigent. Such care is in compliance with the Hospital's mission. Because the Hospital does not pursue collection of amounts determined to qualify as charity care, they are not reported as revenue.

The Hospital maintains records to identify and monitor the level of charity care it provides. These records include the amount of charges forgone for services and supplies furnished under its charity care policy. During the years ended March 31, 2000, and 1999 such charges forgone totaled $395,000 and $375,000, respectively.

NOTE 4—NET PATIENT SERVICE REVENUE

The Hospital provides health care services through its inpatient and outpatient care facilities. The mix of receivables from patients and third-party payers at March 31, 2000, and 1999 is as follows:

	2000	*1999*
Medicare	30.0%	28.5%
Medicaid	15.0	16.0
Patients	13.0	12.5
Other third-party payers	42.0	43.0
Total	100.0%	100.0%

The Hospital has agreements with third-party payers that provide for payments to the Hospital at amounts different from its established rates. Contractual adjustments under third-party reimbursement programs represent the difference between the Hospital's established rates for services and amounts paid by third-party payers. A summary of the payment arrangements with major third-party payers follows:

Medicare. Inpatient acute care rendered to Medicare program beneficiaries is paid at prospectively determined rates-per-discharge. These rates vary according to a patient classification system that is based on clinical, diagnostic, and other factors. Inpatient nonacute care services and certain outpatient services are paid based upon either a cost reimbursement method, established fee screens, or a combination thereof. The Hospital is reimbursed for cost reimbursable items at a tentative rate with final settlement determination after submission of annual cost reports by the Hospital and audits by the Medicare fiscal intermediary. At the current year end, all Medicare settlements for the previous two years are subject to audit and retroactive adjustments.

Medicaid. Inpatient services rendered to Medicaid program beneficiaries are reimbursed at prospectively determined rates-per-day. Outpatient services rendered to Medicaid program beneficiaries are reimbursed at prospectively determined rates-per-visit.

Blue Cross. Inpatient services rendered to Blue Cross subscribers are reimbursed under a cost reimbursement methodology. The Hospital is reimbursed at a tentative rate with final settlement determined after submission of annual cost reports by the Hospital and audits by Blue Cross. The Blue Cross cost report for the prior year end is subject to audit and retroactive adjustment.

The Hospital has also entered into payment agreements with certain commercial insurance carriers, health maintenance organizations, and preferred provider organizations. The bases for payment under these agreements include discounts from established charges and prospectively determined daily rates.

Gross patient service revenue for services rendered by the Hospital under the Medicare, Medicaid, and Blue Cross payment agreements for the years ended March 31, 2000, and 1999 is approximately as follows:

| | 2000 | | 1999 | |
	Amount	*%*	*Amount*	*%*
Medicare	$20,850,000	43.0	$19,900,000	42.0
Medicaid	10,190,000	21.0	10,200,000	21.5
All other payers	17,460,000	36.0	17,300,000	36.5
	$48,500,000	100.0	$47,400,000	100.0

NOTE 5—PROPERTY, PLANT, AND EQUIPMENT

The Hospital's property, plant, and equipment at March 31, 2000, and 1999 are as follows:

	2000	1999
Buildings and improvements	$14,700,000	$14,000,000
Land improvements	1,100,000	1,100,000
Equipment	28,900,000	27,600,000
Total	$44,700,000	$42,700,000

Accumulated depreciation	(26,100,000)	(24,200,000)
Net Depreciable Assets	$18,600,000	$18,500,000
Land	480,000	480,000
Construction in progress	220,000	220,000
Net Property, Plant, Equipment	$19,300,000	$19,200,000

Construction in progress, which involves a renovation project, has not progressed in the last twelve-month period because of a zoning dispute. The project will not require significant outlay to reach completion, as anticipated additional expenditures are currently estimated at $100,000.

NOTE 6—LONG-TERM DEBT

Long-term debt consists of the following:

	2000	*1999*
Hospital Facility Revenue Bonds (Series 1995) at varying interest rates from 4.5% to 5.5%, depending on date of maturity through 2010.	$6,000,000	$6,500,000

The future maturities of long-term debt are as follows:

Years Ending March 31	
1999	$ 475,000
2000	500,000
2001	525,000
2002	550,000
2003	575,000
2004	600,000
Thereafter	3,750,000

Under the terms of the Trust Indenture the following funds (held by the trustee) were established:

Interest Fund

The Hospital deposits (monthly) into the Interest Fund an amount equal to one-sixth of the next semi-annual interest payment due on the bonds.

Bond Sinking Fund

The Hospital deposits (monthly) into the Bond Sinking Fund an amount equal to one-twelfth of the principal due on the next July 1.

Debt Service Reserve Fund

The Debt Service Reserve Fund must be maintained at an amount equal to 10 percent of the aggregate principal amount of all bonds then outstanding. It is to be used to make up any deficiencies in the Interest Fund and Bond Sinking Fund.

Assets held by the trustee under the Trust Indenture at March 31, 2000, and 1999 are as follows:

	2000	1999
Interest Fund	$ 300,000	$ 325,000
Bond Sinking Fund	525,000	500,000
Debt Service Reserve	600,000	650,000
Total	$1,425,000	$1,475,000

NOTE 7—COMMITMENTS

At March 31, 2000, the Hospital had commitments outstanding for a renovation project at the Hospital of approximately $100,000. Construction in progress on the renovation has not progressed in the last twelve-month period because of a zoning dispute. Upon resolution of the dispute, remaining construction costs will be funded from Corporate Funded Depreciation cash reserves.

SOLUTIONS TO PRACTICE EXERCISES

SOLUTION TO PRACTICE EXERCISE 5–I

	Intensive Care Unit	Laboratory	Laundry
Drugs requisitioned	X		
Pathology supplies		X	
Detergents and bleach			X
Nursing salaries	X		
Clerical salaries	X	X	X
Uniforms (for laundry aides)			X
Repairs (parts for microscopes)		X	

Note: If no clerical salaries are assigned to Laundry, this is an acceptable alternative solution.

SOLUTION TO PRACTICE EXERCISE 6–I

	Direct Cost	Indirect Cost
Managed care marketing expense	X	
Real estate taxes		X
Liability insurance		X
Clinic telephone expense	X	
Utilities (for the entire facility)		X
Emergency room medical supplies	X	

SOLUTION TO PRACTICE EXERCISE 6–II

In real life the solution to this exercise will depend upon factors unique to the particular organization. The following solution is a generic one.

	Responsibility Center	Support Center
Security	X	
Communications	X	
Ambulance services	X	
Medical records		X
Educational resources		X
Human resources		X

Reporting: Each Responsibility Center has a manager. All report to the Director.

SOLUTION TO PRACTICE EXERCISE 7–I

Step 1. Find the highest volume of 1,100 packs at a cost of $7,150 in September and the lowest volume of 100 packs at a cost of $1,010 in August.

Step 2. Compute the variable rate per pack as:

	# of Packs	Training Pack Cost
Highest volume	1,100	$7,150
Lowest volume	100	1,010
Difference	1,000	$6,140

Step 3. Divide the difference in cost ($6,140) by the difference in # of packs (1,000) to arrive at the variable cost rate:

$6,140 divided by 1,000 packs = $6.14 per pack

Step 4. Compute the fixed overhead rate as follows:

At the highest level:

Total cost	$7,150
Less: Variable portion [1,100 packs × $6.14 @]	(6,754)
Fixed Portion of Cost	$396

At the lowest level:

Total cost	$1,010
Less: Variable portion [100 packs × $6.14 @]	(614)
Fixed Portion of Cost	$ 396

Proof totals: $396 fixed portion at both levels.

SOLUTION TO PRACTICE EXERCISE 7–II

Step 1. Divide costs into variable and fixed portions. In this case $3,450,000 times 40 percent equals $1,380,000 variable cost and $3,450,000 times 60 percent equals $2,070,000 fixed cost.

Step 2. Compute the contribution margin:

	Amount
Revenue	$3,500,000
Less variable cost	(1,380,000)
Contribution margin	$2,120,000
Less fixed cost	2,070,000
Operating income	$ 50,000

SOLUTION TO PRACTICE EXERCISE 7–III

	Amount	*%*	
Revenue	$1,210,000	100.00	
Less variable cost	(205,000)	16.94	
Contribution margin	$1,005,000	83.06	= PV or CM Ratio
Less fixed cost	(1,100,000)	90.91	
Operating loss	$ (95,000)	7.85	

SOLUTION TO PRACTICE EXERCISE 8–I

1. Compute Net Paid Days Worked

Total days in business year		364
Less two days off per week		104
# Paid days per year		260
Less paid days not worked		
Holidays	8	
Sick days	5	
Education day	1	
Vacation days	5	
		19
Net paid days worked		241

2. Convert Net Paid Days Worked to a Factor

Total days in business year divided by net paid days worked equals factor

364/241 = 1.510373

SOLUTION TO PRACTICE EXERCISE 8–II

	Shift 1 Day	Shift 2 Evening	Shift 3 Night	=	24-Hour Scheduling Total
Position: Admissions officer	2	1	1		4 8-hour shifts
FTEs—to cover position					
7 days/week equals	2.8	1.4	1.4		5.6 FTEs
Position: Clerical	1	0	0		1 8-hour shift
FTEs—to cover position					
7 days/week equals	1.4	0	0		1.4 FTEs

SOLUTION TO PRACTICE EXERCISE 9–I

Common sizing for the assets of the two hospitals appears on the worksheet below. Note that their gross numbers are very different, yet the proportionate relationships of the percentages (20 percent, 75 percent, and 5 percent) are the same for both hospitals.

	Same Year for Both Hospitals			
	Hospital A		*Hospital B*	
Current assets	$ 2,000,000	20%	$ 8,000,000	20%
Property, plant, and equipment	7,500,000	75%	30,000,000	75%
Other assets	500,000	5%	2,000,000	5%
Total assets	$10,000,000	100%	$40,000,000	100%

SOLUTION TO PRACTICE EXERCISE 9–II

		Hospital A		
	Year 1	*Year 2*	*Difference*	
Current assets	$1,600,000	$ 2,000,000	$ 400,000	25%
Property, plant, and equipment	6,000,000	7,500,000	1,500,000	25%
Other assets	400,000	500,000	100,000	25%
Total assets	$8,000,000	$10,000,000	$2,000,000	—

Note: The worksheet below shows Hospital A with both common sizing and trend analysis:

		Hospital A				
	Year 1		*Year 2*		*Difference*	
Current assets	$1,600,000	20%	$ 2,000,000	20%	$ 400,000	25%
Property, plant, and equipment	6,000,000	75%	7,500,000	75%	1,500,000	25%
Other assets	400,000	5%	500,000	5%	100,000	25%
Total assets	$8,000,000	100%	$10,000,000	100%	$2,000,000	—

SOLUTION TO PRACTICE EXERCISE 10–I

Your initial budget assumptions were as follows:

Assume the budget anticipated 30,000 inpatient days this year at an average of $650 revenue per day, or $19,500,000. Further assume that inpatient expenses were budgeted at $600 per patient day, or $18,000,000. Also assume the budget anticipated 10,000 outpatient visits this year at an average of $400 revenue per visit, or $4,000,000. Further assume that outpatient expenses were budgeted at $380 per visit, or $3,800,000. The budget worksheet would look like this:

	As Budgeted
Revenue—Inpatient	$19,500,000
Revenue—Outpatient	4,000,000
Subtotal	$23,500,000
Expenses—Inpatient	$18,000,000
Expenses—Outpatient	3,800,000
Subtotal	$21,800,000
Excess of revenue over expenses	$1,700,000

Now assume that only 27,000, or 90 percent, of the patient days are going to actually be achieved for the year. The average revenue of $650 per day will be achieved for these 27,000 days (thus 27,000 times 650 equals 17,550,000). Also assume that outpatient visits will actually amount to 110 percent, or 11,000 for the year. The average revenue of $400 per visit will be achieved for these 11,000 visits (thus 11,000 times 400 equals 4,400,000). Further assume that, due to the heroic efforts of the Chief Financial Officer, the actual inpatient expenses will amount to $11,600,000 and the actual outpatient expenses will amount to $4,000,000. The actual results would look like this:

	Actual
Revenue—Inpatient	$17,550,000
Revenue—Outpatient	4,400,000
Subtotal	$21,950,000
Expenses—Inpatient	16,100,000
Expenses—Outpatient	4,000,000
Subtotal	$20,100,000
Excess of revenue over expenses	$1,850,000

Since the budgeted revenues and expenses still reflect the original expectations of 30,000 inpatient days and 10,000 outpatient visits, the budget report would look like this:

	Actual	*Budget*	*Static Budget Variance*
Revenue—Inpatient	$17,550,000	$19,500,000	$(1,950,000)
Revenue—Outpatient	4,400,000	4,000,000	400,000
Subtotal	$21,950,000	$23,500,000	$(1,550,000)
Expenses—Inpatient	$16,100,000	$18,000,000	$(1,900,000)
Expenses—Outpatient	4,000,000	3,800,000	200,000
Subtotal	$20,100,000	$21,800,000	$(1,700,000)
Excess of revenue over expenses	$ 1,850,000	$ 1,700,000	$ 150,000

Note: The negative effect of the $1,550,000 net drop in revenue is offset by the greater effect of the $1,700,000 net drop in expenses, resulting in a positive net effect of $150,000.

REQUIRED SOLUTION TO PRACTICE EXERCISE 10–II

The Price Variance is $206,100 (3,435,000 less 3,228,900 equals 206,100).
The Quantity Variance is $185,000 (3,435,000 less 3,250,000 equals 185,000).

OPTIONAL SOLUTION TO PRACTICE EXERCISE 10–II

The $3,228,900 actual overhead costs represent 687,000 RVUs times $4.70 per RVU.
The $3,250,000 budgeted overhead costs represent 650,000 RVUs times $5.00 per RVU.

SOLUTION TO PRACTICE EXERCISE 11–I: UNADJUSTED RATE OF RETURN

1. Calculation using original investment amount:

$$\frac{\$100,000}{\$500,000} = 20\% \text{ Unadjusted Rate of Return}$$

2. Calculation using average investment amount:

First Step: Compute average investment amount for total unrecovered asset cost:

At beginning of estimated useful life = $500,000
At end of estimated useful life   = $ <u>50,000</u>
   Sum $550,000
Divided by 2 = $275,000 average investment amount

Second Step: Calculate unadjusted rate of return:

$$\frac{\$100,000}{\$275,000} = 36.4\% \text{ Unadjusted Rate of Return}$$

SOLUTION TO PRACTICE EXERCISE 11–II: FINDING THE FUTURE VALUE (WITH A COMPOUND INTEREST TABLE)

Step 1. Refer to the Compound Interest Table found in Appendix 11–B at the back of this chapter. Reading across, or horizontally, find the 7 percent column. Reading down, or vertically, find Year 6. Trace across the Year 6 line item to the 7 percent column. The factor is 1.501.

Step 2. Multiply the current savings account balance of $11,000 times the factor of 1.501 to find the future value of $16,511. In six years at compound interest of 7 percent, the college fund will have a balance of $16,511.

SOLUTION TO PRACTICE EXERCISE 11–III: FINDING THE PRESENT VALUE

Step 1. Refer to the Present Value Table found in Appendix 11–A at the back of this chapter. Reading across, or horizontally, find the 7 percent column. Reading down, or vertically, find Year 15. Trace across the Year 15 line item to the 7 percent column. The factor is 0.3624.

Step 2. Multiply $150,000 times the factor of 0.3624 to find the present value of $54,360.

SOLUTION TO PRACTICE EXERCISE 11–IV

Assemble the assumptions in an orderly manner:

Assumption 1: Initial cost of the investment = $16,950.
Assumption 2: Estimated annual net cash inflow the investment will generate = $3,000.
Assumption 3: Useful life of the asset = 10 years.

Perform calculation:

Step 1: Divide the initial cost of the investment ($16,950) by the estimated annual net cash inflow it will generate ($3,000). The answer is a ratio amounting to 5.650.
Step 2: Now use the abbreviated look-up table for the Present Value of an Annuity of $1, which is found at the back of the Examples and Exercises section. Find the line item for the number of periods that matches the useful life of the asset (10 years in this case).
Step 3: Look across the 10 year line on the table and find the column that approximates the ratio of 5.650 (as computed in Step 1). That column contains the interest rate representing the rate of return. In this case the rate of return is 12 percent.

SOLUTION TO PRACTICE EXERCISE 11–V

Assemble assumptions in an orderly manner:

Assumption 1: Purchase price of the equipment = $500,000.
Assumption 2: Useful life of the equipment = 10 years.
Assumption 3: Revenue the machine will generate per year = $84,000.
Assumption 4: Direct operating costs associated with earning the revenue = $21,000.
Assumption 5: Depreciation expense per year (computed as purchase price per assumption 1 divided by useful life per assumption 2) = $50,000.

Perform computation:

Step 1: Find the machine's expected net income after taxes:

Revenue (Assumption 3)		$84,000
Less		
Direct operating costs (Assumption 4)	$21,000	
Depreciation (Assumption 5)	50,000	
		71,000
Net income		$13,000

Note: No income taxes for this hospital.

Step 2: Find the net annual cash inflow the machine is expected to generate (in other words, convert the net income to a cash basis).

Net income	$13,000
Add back depreciation (a noncash expenditure)	50,000
Annual net cash inflow after taxes	$63,000

Step 3: Compute the payback period:

$$\frac{\text{Investment}}{\text{Net annual cash inflow}} = \frac{\$500,000 \text{ machine cost *}}{\$63,000} = 7.9 \text{ year payback period}$$

*assumption 1 above
**per Step 2 above

The machine will pay back its investment under these assumptions in 7⁹⁄₁₀ years.

SOLUTION TO PRACTICE EXERCISE 12–I

Current Liabilities	30,000
Total Assets	1,000,000
Income from Operations	80,000
Accumulated Depreciation	480,000
Total Operating Revenue	180,000
Current Portion of Long-Term Debt	10,000
Interest Income	-0-
Inventories	5,000

SOLUTION TO PRACTICE EXERCISE 12–II

1. Straight-line depreciation would amount to $54,000 per year for 10 years. This amount is computed as follows:
   Step 1. Compute the cost net of salvage or trade-in value: 600,000 less 10 percent salvage value or 60,000 equals 540,000.
   Step 2. Divide the resulting figure by the expected life (also known as estimated useful life): 540,000 divided by 10 equals 54,000 depreciation per year for 10 years.

2. Double declining depreciation is computed as follows:
   Step 1. Compute the straight-line rate: 1 divided by 10 equals 10 percent.
   Step 2. Now double the rate (as in "double declining method"): 10 percent times 2 equals 20 percent.
   Step 3. Compute the first year's depreciation expense: 600,000 times 20 percent = 120,000.
   Step 4. Compute the carry-forward book value at the beginning of the second year: 600,000 book value beginning Year 1 less Year 1 depreciation of 120,000 equals book value at beginning of the second year of 480,000.
   Step 5. Compute the second year's depreciation expense: 480,000 times 20 percent = 96,000.
   Step 6. Compute the carry-forward book value at the beginning of the third year: 480,000 book value beginning Year 2 less Year 2 depreciation of 96,000 equals book value at beginning of the third year of 384,000.

—Continue until the asset's salvage or trade-in value has been reached.

Book Value at Beginning of Year	Depreciation Expense	Book Value at End of Year
600,000	600,000 × 20% = 120,000	600,000 – 120,000 = 480,000
480,000	480,000 × 20% = 96,000	480,000 – 96,000 = 384,000
384,000	384,000 × 20% = 76,800	384,000 – 76,800 = 307,200
307,200	307,200 × 20% = 61,440	307,200 – 61,440 = 245,760
245,760	245,760 × 20% = 49,152	245,760 – 49,152 = 196,608
196,608	196,608 × 20% = 39,322	196,608 – 39,322 = 157,286
157,286	157,286 × 20% = 31,457	157,286 – 31,457 = 125,829
125,829	125,829 × 20% = 25,166	125,829 – 25,166 = 100,663
100,663	100,663 × 20% = 20,132	100,663 – 20,132 = 80,531
80,531	80,561 at 10th year:	80,561 – 20,561 = 60,000

—Balance remaining at end of tenth year represents the salvage or trade-in value.

Note: Under the double declining balance method, book value never reaches zero. Therefore, a company typically adopts the straight-line method at the point where straight line would exceed the double declining balance.

SOLUTION TO PRACTICE EXERCISE 13–I

Current Ratio

The current ratio is represented as Current Ratio = Current Assets divided by Current Liabilities. This ratio is considered to be a measure of short-term debt-paying ability. However, it must be carefully interpreted.

Current Ratio Computation

$$\frac{\text{Current Assets}}{\text{Current Liabilities}} = \frac{\$70,000}{\$30,000} = 2.33 \text{ to } 1$$

Quick Ratio

The quick ratio is represented as Quick Ratio = Cash + Short-Term Investments + Net Receivables divided by Current Liabilities. This ratio is considered to be an even more severe test of short-term debt-paying ability (even more severe than the current ratio). The quick ratio is also known as the acid-test ratio, for obvious reasons.

$$\frac{\text{Cash \& Cash Equivalents} + \text{Net Receivables}}{\text{Current Liabilities}} = \frac{\$65,000}{\$30,000} = 2.167 \text{ to } 1$$

SOLUTION TO PRACTICE EXERCISE 13–II

Solvency Ratios

Debt Service Coverage Ratio (DSCR)

The Debt Service Coverage Ratio (DSCR) is represented as change in unrestricted net assets (net income) plus interest, depreciation, and amortization divided by maximum annual debt service. This ratio is universally used in credit analysis, and figures prominently in the Mini-Case Study #1.

$$\frac{\text{Change in Unrestricted Net Assets (net income)}}{\text{plus Interest, Depreciation, Amortization}} = \frac{\$113,100}{\$22,200} = 5.1$$

Note: $80,000 + $3,100 + $30,000 = $113,100.

Liabilities To Fund Balance (or Debt to Net Worth)

The liabilities to fund balance or net worth computation is represented as total liabilities divided by unrestricted net assets (fund balances)(or net worth) = total debt divided by tangible net worth. This figure is a quick indicator of debt load.

$$\frac{\text{Total Liabilities}}{\text{Unrestricted Fund Balances}} = \frac{\$200,000}{\$800,000} = 2.5$$

SOLUTION TO PRACTICE EXERCISE 13–III

Profitability Ratios

Operating Margin

The operating margin, which is generally expressed as a percentage, is represented as operating income (loss) divided by total operating revenues. This ratio is used for a number of managerial purposes and also sometimes enters into credit analysis. It is therefore a multi-purpose measure.

$$\frac{\text{Operating Income (Loss)}}{\text{Total Operating Revenues}} = \frac{\$80,000}{\$180,000} = 44.4\%$$

Return on Total Assets

The return on total assets is represented as earnings before interest and taxes (EBIT) divided by total assets. This is a broad measure in common use.

$$\frac{\text{EBIT (Earnings Before Interest \& Taxes)}}{\text{Total Assets}} = \frac{\$83,100}{\$1,000,000} = 8.3\%$$

Note: $80,000 + $3,100 = $83,100.

Index

About the Authors

Judith J. Baker, PhD, CPA, is Executive Director of Resource Group, Ltd., a Dallas-based health care consulting firm. She earned her Bachelor of Science degree in Business Administration at the University of Missouri, Columbia and her Master of Liberal Studies with a concentration in Business Management at the University of Oklahoma, Norman. She earned her Master of Arts and Doctorate in Human and Organizational Systems, with a concentration in costing systems, at the Fielding Institute, Santa Barbara, California. She is an adjunct faculty member at the Case Western Reserve University Frances Payne Bolton School of Nursing.

Judith has over thirty years experience in health care and consults on numerous health care systems and costing problems. She has worked with health care systems, costing, and reimbursement throughout her career. As a HCFA subcontractor she assists in validation of costs for new programs and for rate setting and consults on cost report design.

Judith has written over 40 articles, manuals, and books. She is Consulting Editor for Aspen Publishers, Inc. Her latest books are *Activity-Based Costing and Activity-Based Management for Health Care, Prospective Payment for Long-Term Care: An Annual Guide,* and *Prospective Payment for Home Health Agencies* (all Aspen publications). She is co-editor of the quarterly *Journal of Healthcare Finance.*

R.W. Baker, JD, is Managing Partner of Resource Group, Ltd., a Dallas-based health care consulting firm. He has more than 30 years of experience in health care and has designed, directed, and administered numerous financial impact studies for health care providers. His recent studies have centered around facility-specific MDS data collection and analysis. He and his firm have subcontracted to the HCFA Nursing Home Case Mix and Quality Demonstration from 1990 to present.

R.W. is the editor of continuing professional education seminar manuals and training manuals for facility personnel and for research staff members. He is a Consulting Editor with Aspen Publishers, Inc. and is co-author of *A Step-by-Step Guide to the Minimum Data Set* (Aspen Publishers, Inc. 1999).